N

Radiant Skin Care Secrets & Homemade Beauty Recipes from the World's Most Unforgettable Women

Elizabeth Fellow

Elizabeth Fellow

Table of Contents

Introduction

Beauty has turned a corner. We have gone back to our roots. The savvy woman understands she does not have to spend thousands of dollars on skin care to get amazing results, but just because she's not supporting the beauty industry doesn't mean she can't have amazingly luxurious creations with which to adorn herself.

For thousands of years, women and their attendants have blended, experimented, and concocted custom products to suit their needs, healing the skin, the body, the emotions, and even the mind.

Within these pages you too will learn the secrets of how to use precious stones to nourish your skin, essential oils to soothe and heal, and fruits and soils to cleanse and detoxify.

Discover why your skin is dry or how to get rid of blackheads for good. For the days when the zipper on your jeans refuses to shut, there's even a remedy for that. An inch off the hips... in 20 minutes flat... seriously!

You'll even learn how to make an edible chocolate body cream infused with gold-leaf to indulge in with your lover.

This is no ordinary natural beauty book. Looking through the lens of history at some of the most unforgettable women the world has ever seen, it explores their secrets and how you can bring a bit of their lives into your own. It's opulent and opinionated, sage and sexy, with easy-to-follow recipes for newcomers to natural healing and professionals alike.

This is a book whose time has come. A friend of mine dreamed up the concept, and I gleefully rubbed my hands at the idea of a book which was both an introduction to the natural healing forces of the earth I love so dearly, and a celebration of the sisterhood which is our birth right as women.

Lavish creams, luscious oils, unforgettable women, what could be simpler?

Well, as it turned out, splitting the atom might have been an easier option for me.

Some books write themselves, others have a far more difficult labouring.

This one was a stubborn mule which refused to be led where I pleased, but then that's really no surprise. We're not dealing with simpering maids and bland beauties in this book. These women are firebrands, women of power and passion, women of intellect, and yes, great beauty. I was trying to figure out how to tell their stories and their secrets, it was agonising…

Then, a different conversation elapsed in another corner of my life, and I wrote the words "Physician, heal thyself".

So I did.

I raided my box of essential oils to scent my bath and took some valerian tablets to help me sleep. As I waited for my drowsiness to arrive, I whiled away precious moments reading one more research paper than perhaps I should have. Sipping a glass of locally distilled brandy, designed to blow your head off, I did what you really should *not* do, combining the plant from which Valium is derived with a glass of strong alcohol.

An idiot's choice!

Needless to say, once in bed I drifted off into a deliciously deep slumber.

And then the dream began.

Half way between wakefulness and sleep, a very strange scene played through my head.

I watched, amazed, as the book which refused to be written, seemed to fall into place. As my mind wrote… it continued to drift.

Curiouser and curiouser! cried Alice….

The effects of the brandy, the valerian, and the thoughts about the previous day's struggle with the book all unravelled in my sleep. The brandy didn't just blow my head off…

It blew my mind.

To make this book easier to understand, I have broken it into three main sections.

Part 1 takes you into what was essentially the dream I had. "The Spa That Time Forgot," as I have now come to call it, walks you through parallels between the beauty recipes I have created for you and ideas of how they might also have helped some of our most unforgettable women throughout history.

In Part 2, I outline the parts different ingredients play in Natural Beauty so you can begin to get a handle on which ingredients are best for you. First comes a cursory note about the history of natural beauty through the ages. Next I introduce the healing components of a natural beauty regime. Readers of my last book, *Nature's Medicine: The Everyday Guide to Herbal Remedies & Healing Recipes for Common Ailments*, will be familiar with the fruits and some of the essential oils, but to this I have added a section about blending precious stones and metals into treatments, as well as a look at healing clays too.

In Part 3, I outline the beauty recipes we explored in The Spa and how to prepare them. These are separated from the narrative, for your ease of use.

This book is a strange and wonderful journey down the rabbit hole and through one of my most bizarre dreams. It's quirky, and catty, with more than a little bit of a madness thrown in.

As Aristotle said, **"No great mind has ever existed without a touch of madness."**

At least that's what I like to tell myself!

You decide.

Whatever your thoughts, I hope you enjoy the ride!

As you close your eyes, you are taken through your spa treatments by the rather dishy (if not, at times, a little campy) Alchemist. His are the hands which blend your creams and smooth them over your skin.

It's important that you try not to get too distracted by his pearly white teeth, and you listen carefully to what he has to say. His knowledge is in skin care and beauty, and plants and crystals, and he teaches you to create the most remarkable things.

It seems it is no mistake you have arrived today at The Spa, for The Alchemist works at the bidding of a strange and enigmatic woman you will come to know as The Healer.

Unlike the serene White Witch you might associate with the healing arts, The Healer is a more "earthy" type, who fancies herself a bit of an epochal vigilante, righting wrongs of the past as she sees them, protecting the women who need her, and slapping the occasional diva indulging in a temper tantrum.

You will see the world as it has unfolded through *her* eyes.

Some of the women you meet you may love; other's maybe not so much. You may learn a lot about where your own character comes from as The Healer shows you womanhood, glorious warts and all.

The Healer may have a short temper and a flirtatious edge, but like all women, there is more to her than meets the eye. She is a wise, wise woman with a great knowledge of what nature can do. Hidden in her treatments there is always a message to "treat" the woman she visits. Using plants and crystals she shows you other ways you can naturally affect a person's mind, body, and spirit.

Where The Alchemist treats the skin, The Healer has the capacity to influence mental processing, emotional, and physical healing, and as a result help you discover your very Soul.

But the question remains…. why has The Healer picked you?

Part 1

When you reach the "The Spa That Time Forgot," the receptionist greets you and shows you where to go to prepare yourself. As you enter the changing room there is a table set with an ornate silver tea pot and a pretty china tea cup and saucer. Besides the cup is a note with the instruction....

Drink me!

As you swallow the bitter aperitif, you feel a strange and warming glow. Just as you begin to feel a little disoriented, an attendant enters the room.

"What is it?" you ask.

"A drink," he replies with a shrug. "Something to help you remember who you are."

Instinctively you seem to know you're about to explore other lives left behind. Through many incarnations you will remember who you have been and therefore who you have the power to become again.

You sense a difference in you; a knowing. Something you have always known but perhaps have not yet been able to express, something just out of reach...

The handsome man who collects you from the changing rooms takes you in for your treatments to begin.

"I am The Alchemist," he says. "I create the most magical things to help you transform into the beautiful butterfly you are meant to be..." and he flashes a set of pearly white teeth.

He leads you to a deep warm tub and tells you about the creation he is about to add.

The moment you smell or experience any of the treatments, you are transported to a magical corridor with many, many doors where you catch glimpses of The Healer.

You walk along, knowing whichever door she chooses will take her through to a lifetime where she might have used the bounty of the earth to help another great woman before, and you wait with baited breath.

The Alchemist describes a rich nourishing bath, designed to relax you and pamper.

You watch as he mixes, and you understand just how easy it will be to make at home. You smile languorously as he adds the sweet smelling oils, and the water turns a milky white.

As you lie back, your journey begins.

The Healer walks along the corridor. She seems familiar with this place and walks confidently up to a rich wooden door decorated with ornate glyphs of papyrus. In her hand is a beautiful alabaster amphora. She opens the door ….

31 BC Cleopatra

The Healer attends the bath of the woman who she believes may quite possibly be the most beautiful woman the world has ever seen. Well, the menfolk certainly seem to think so, she thinks wryly to herself, as she crosses the room to the bath.

The bath chamber is filled with attendants scurrying around, waiting for their queen. The Healer adds her <u>precious mix of Milk, Rose, and Myrrh</u>, and the room fills with echoes of ooo and aaah as the scent permeates the room.

The Healer wonders to herself, if what they say is true. Could it be that Cleopatra would truly be the last Pharaoh of Egypt? Perhaps it would be so. Cleopatra's Ptolomeic Dynasty had refused to speak Egyptian, instead only Greek, so proud they were of their descent from Alexander the Great. It had made them too accessible to the world, she feared. Now those wretched Romans seemed to be banging the door down to take over.

Her queen was a clever strategist, make no mistake. Consummating a relationship with the Emperor Caesar had ensured she was elevated quickly to the Egyptian throne. She was a steely politician, and her people only loved her more for it. While many people suggested this was because of her beauty, The Healer felt it was more that she just intuitively understood showmanship. Cleopatra seemed instinctively to know how to push a powerful man's buttons to get what she wanted.

The Healer remembered a time the queen had been sailing down the Nile, her flotilla behind her, and she (The Healer) and the other attendants of the bath chamber had strewn thousands and thousands of rose petals off the bow of the barge. As the petals floated on the surface of the Nile, baking in the warm African sun, the most gloriously heady scent filled the air. The effects were nothing short of sorcery. Was it Cleopatra's beauty the people worshipped, perhaps, The Healer laughed to herself, or more likely were they pleasantly drugged by her presence?

The Healer knew her own place was prized above all others in the household since   people whispered the richness of Cleopatra's pale complexion was made even lovelier by an elixir The Healer had created. The queen religiously bathed in her milk bath every day. Redolent of precious oils, her skin was made rich and smooth by the protein from asses' milk.

That poor woman, in 44 B.C., when her husband Caesar was murdered, Cleopatra had been beyond furious. The Healer recalled how she had so cleverly aligned herself with Mark Anthony in a bid to overthrow her loathed opponent, Gaius Julius Caesar Octavianus. The Healer had wanted to throttle Octavianus for upsetting her queen. Often she had thought about giving him a piece of her mind, but backed off when she imagined how foolish she would look when she couldn't get his name out!

Now she adored seeing her queen so happy as Mark Anthony headed off to battle tomorrow in the hope of defeating her foe.

As the queen entered the bath chamber, The Healer bowed and then left the room through the door from whence she came.

When you see The Healer would you tell her?

Sadly that next day was the beginning of the end for her beloved queen and in turn, the reign of the great Egyptian Pharoahs. After being beaten in battle by Octavian, Mark Anthony committed suicide. Tragically, the beautiful Cleopatra followed suit. She was, they say, bitten by an asp. The Healer might also find it interesting to hear it is thanks to Cleopatra's love for Greek we are now able to translate hieroglyphics. The Rosetta stone, written in both languages, held the key.

Cleopatra 69-30 BC

****

You rouse from the reverie of <u>Cleopatra's Milk Bath with Rose Petal and Myrrh</u> as the alchemist calls your name.

You open your eyes and he asks "Ready to remember more?"

You nod, and he leads you to another, more humble looking, bath.

"This time we will use only oils," he says. It is wonderful for days when you are too stressed with the responsibility of being a mother, or career woman, or even sister, daughter, or aunt….and you just want to have a little bit if "Me time" and remember who you are.

He adds <u>"Remember Who I am" Bath Oil </u>to your tub.

As you lie back and ease your shoulders into the water, you relax, excited for the elixir to show you more.

Jerusalem, 30 AD

The Healer finds herself outside a door fashioned out of rough stone, less a door really, than a cleft between the rocks. As she wriggles herself through the gap, she braces herself for one of the hardest things she has had to do in any of her lives. Before her are a small group of women

16

around a stone that marks the closure of a tomb. Wailing, they lament the crucifixion of the man these women believe to be the Son of God.

The Healer knows these women well, especially the two called Mary. Today she is here to help the mother. The Healer sits, with her jar of oils ready, waiting for the correct moment to pass them on. For many an hour she watches, beneath the hot baking sun.

Scorched by the temperature of the midday sun, Mary, Mother of God, eventually throws off her mantle and lays it on the large shrub beside her. The Healer watches as the blue robe touches the white flowers of the rosemary bush and changes their hue. The Healer wistfully recalls in every later life when she has chosen the plant, its flowers had remained the colours of Mary's coat.

Finally, the bereaved mother cries the words The Healer had known would eventually come.

"If I am not His mother, then what in heaven's name am I?"

Every mother ultimately faces the realisation of an empty nest, some more tragically than others, and must remember who she truly is.

Quietly, The Healer walks over to the bush, and places her small jar on top of Mary's coat. She knows this will help her remember just who she is; the rosemary to aid memory, the frankincense to instil confidence, and the myrrh to ground and heal.

Then The Healer disappears again, through the cleft in the rocks.

Mary of Galilee 20 BC-41 AD

****

The alchemist waits patiently for you to come back. When you open your eyes, he asks carefully "Are you OK?" You nod sadly, and he seems to understand where you have been.

Next he describes how he is going to make an exfoliating facial Massage Treatment for you and mixes <u>Margo Fonteyn's Hazelnut and Camellia Exfoliating Facial Massage Oil</u>.

The Healer knows this door well, and she holds her posy of Camellia flowers and hazel branches in her hand for just a moment longer. Looking down at the flowers, she listens to the enigmatic sound of the rehearsal the other side of the door. The light and melancholy notes of Chopin's La Dame aux Camellia never fail to move her.

As she walks through the door she enters…

1964 back stage at The Royal Ballet Company with Margot Fonteyn.

Before an empty auditorium, the dancer they were calling the greatest ballerina of all time, Margot Fonteyn practices her legendary foutté pirouettes. Many times The Healer asked her how she managed to not to get dizzy. No matter how many times Margot had explained it, she never quite understood how "spotting" worked.

"I am glad I don't get it," thinks The Healer "It would be like understanding how they pull a rabbit out of the hat… it would kill the magic."

The Healer steals discretely through to Madame's changing room and lays her posy down. She checks that she has enough marigold and myrrh balm to relieve the blisters from the ballerina's pointes after the show, and refills the lavender and juniper muscle rub too.

Fonteyn had told The Healer many stories of how, as a child of 8, her family had moved from their home in Surrey, England to China for her father's work.

In Shanghai, she had met a Russian émigré, George Gonchorov, who had cemented her love of ballet.

When she had returned in to England in 1933, at the age of 14, she had secured a place at the Vic-Wells Ballet (the forerunner to the Royal Ballet) and trained under the immortal Ninette de Valois.

Whilst most people lauded Fonteyn's Aurora from Sleeping Beauty the most, The Healer had her own special preference. The posy was a secret joke between them. Before each new production, The Healer would attach a symbol to a hazel branch (a symbol of her love of the nutcracker) to ask the ballerina, can you match this?

Her job done, smiling, The Healer leaves the room and heads for her place in the stall to watch Fonteyn and Nureyev perform in one of the greatest partnerships the world would ever see.

When Fonteyn enters her dressing room, she notices the camellia flower and the requisite hazel twigs, and she smiles, grateful for the support and friendship of the woman who cares for her health.

Margot Fonteyn: 1919-1991

****

On your return to the spa, the Alchemist confides, "Her Aurora was without parallel," as he sashays across to the herb cupboard again.

This time, he explains, he will use an amber elixir, made from fossilized tree resin over 20,000 years old, combined with Oakmoss as a deep cleanser.

Mixing that with pear and watermelon to hydrate the skin, and banana to give it a delicious nourishing edge, he says, "It's cooling, and you can almost feel the grime being pulled to the surface!"

As the oils of <u>Lucrezia Borgia's Deep Cleaning Mask</u>, begin to soak in, you sense The Healer coming to you, but she is not her usual tranquil self.....

1502 Vatican City

The Healer supposed it should be the place where God dwelt, but she highly doubted it. Through her many incarnations, she felt the Vatican might have enjoyed better days, to say the least.

Here in the renaissance papacy of Pope Alexander VI, Machiavellian politics and sexual corruption was about all she could see. And right in the middle of it was the Pope's daughter, Lucrezia.

It was hard to say just how complicit the girl was in the evil wrangling of the day. What was certain was that this was not the first marriage which had been arranged for her with power in mind. No, in fact this was number three, and The Healer didn't want to consider whether all the rumours of dalliances were true.

God-fearing house? The Healer wasn't so sure.

She thought it was probably Lucrezia's beauty to blame. Blonde hair past her knees, hazel eyes which changed colour with her moods, a high bosom, and grace which made her appear to walk on air....

No wonder the men folk all seemed to fall for her.

The Borgia girl certainly knew how to make the best of that long slender neck, adorning it with all manner of opulent jewels. The Healer laid down her latest acquisition; a long strand of amber beads to be worn as a protection from evil.

As The Healer left the room she mused, "With the trouble that girl gets into, another protective amulet isn't going to hurt...."

1480-1519 Lucrezia Borgia

The alchemist says nothing, rather he raises a disapproving eyebrow and shakes his head.

He asks if you are ready to see how to make a cleansing lotion. You nod and are excited to hear what wondrously precious ingredients he will use.

"Carrots," you say disappointedly "The best you can find is carrots....?"

He reassures you that Jessica Rabbit's Carrot and Orange Cleansing Lotion is the best detoxifier you will find. You watch as he shows you how to blend it.

The carrot will lift any dirt and debris from the skin, but it is also a tonic for the liver, the organ which controls the entire bodily detoxification system. The orange is refining, and the cypress and grapefruit get right down into the pores to clean them thoroughly.

The Healer knew she was about to come face to face with madness. Stepping through, she burst through the wall of

Jessica Rabbit's Toon Town Warehouse

As The Healer checked herself out, she was pretty pleased with this Technicolor line drawing version of herself. Far better than any other incarnation, she thought; although, she would admit to wishing for a smidgen more shading at the cheekbones. Still, she couldn't complain.

*The dame she was about to meet, however; now she really **did** get the luck of the draw!*

Lustrous red hair flopping over heavy lids, a tiny button nose almost invisible next to her blood-red pout... you'd think that was enough, but no, you saw Jessica Rabbit's face... later!

Of course, every one said she was guilty of framing her beloved husband Roger, but The Healer wouldn't believe it. Couldn't believe it! The rabbit was certainly nothing short of obsessed with the singer, but Mrs. Rabbit utterly adored her husband.

It was right too, what Jessica had said to that Detective, "I'm not bad, I'm just drawn that way!"

She did look like bad news but Jessica was a loyal and sincere wife just looking to make a buck. Sure, her singing gig at The Los Angeles Supper Club wasn't the kind of job you would normally associate with a respectable woman, but a girl's gotta live!

The Healer walked into the club and approached the stage where the auburn beauty rehearsed. She handed over a bunch of carrots "A bit of something for Roger to let him know I am thinking of him."

A heavy eye shaded in purple shimmer winked a heartfelt thank you.

The Healer skipped out, turned to wave, and thought... yep, Jessica definitely got better shading!

When you see The Healer let her know...
In 2008, Jessica Rabbit was selected by Empire Magazine as one of The 100 Greatest Movie Characters of All Time

Jessica Krupnick-Rabbit, 1988 – Present

****

You come to giggling. The Alchemist reaches over and shoos away the cartoon bluebird that's followed you back.

"Ready for madness of a different kind?" he asks. "Let's freshen you up!"

Orange flower water fills the air as he shows you how to create Twiggy's Petitgrain Toner to cleanse and refresh your skin. The secret to great-looking skin, he explains, is to always close the pores so that new dirt can't get in. The witch hazel seals them shut and brings the blood supply to the surface.

A little light-headed with the freshness of the blend, you imagine yourself somewhere far away...

London, Carnaby Street 1966:
The Healer loved the feeling of the breeze upon her thighs. There weren't many incarnations in which she got to wear a skirt so short! She mused that perhaps she could do with exposing them to just a little more sun!

London was rockin',man, and she felt absolutely at home, although she had to admit she was selling more herbs for smoking than for making creams lately! Still, baby, this time was groovy!

She laughed again at the coincidence of the cream she was delivering. Petitgrain... made from the twigs and branches of the orange tree, going to the girl

Twiggy, 1966's British Woman of The Year.

Yep, '66 was definitely Twiggy's year.

The Healer had to admit though, it was refreshing to see a different type of beauty rule the covers of the fashion pages. Androgynous physique, huge doe eyes, and short cropped hair, it was a long way from Lucrezia Borgia's dangling tresses and ample bust, that was for sure.

Of course, The Healer knew Twiggy's star would soon burn out. These models always did. They never lasted very long!

"Enjoy it while you can," she thought.

The Healer dropped the Petitgrain concoction, blended to sooth the model's nerves, into the studio office and continued on her way.

When you see The Healer, please tell her....

In 2012, at the age of 62, Lesley Lawson, the model also known as Twiggy, launched her own exclusive clothing label and fronted the English Marks and Spencer TV advertising campaign in a deal reputed to be well over a £1m. She is a fervent campaigner for breast cancer awareness, animal welfare, and is passionately anti-fur. It seems that Twiggy's star never did burn out!

Leslie Hornby Lawson (Twiggy) 1949-Present

****

The alchemist looks and declares, "Refreshing isn't it?" This one is a cooling mask. The aloe vera is like ice when you put it on, and it is very hydrating to the skin. The angelica refines the pores, and the cypress and dill are cleansing.

He applies <u>Joan Of Arc's Cooling Face Mask from the Angels</u>.

As The Healer stands before the courtroom door, she knows she has to be strong. The maiden needs her help, and she is determined to give it. Hard as it is, she has to keep her mouth shut! These are dangerous times to be friends with the girl they are calling "The heretic!"

1431 Outside of the prison cell of Jeanne d'Arc (Joan of Arc)

The Healer was so mad she could spit! She could not believe how the church had sold out her young friend. The cowards were happy enough to let Jeanne head off to battle while they stayed safe in their vestry rooms, but now, when she needed their support, they betrayed her.

She was a good girl... guided by God... or so she believed, anyway. Who was The Healer to argue otherwise?

The Maid of Orleans had been resolute in her assertion that God had told her to take up the cause of Charles VII to regain France from the hands of the English.
She had done everything she had been asked to do. How could this end with her being burned at the stake? The Healer knew what being guided by God could do for you.... It seemed not so many lifetimes since she had hidden before the Christ's tomb, watching His mother.

Jeanne, the daughter of peasants, had been a young girl of 14 when, she believed, she was visited by the Archangel Michael and told to fight in what became known as the 100 Years War. Guided by her angels, she took up arms for Charles VII, the Dauphin of France. After lifting a siege in just nine days, the soon-to-be-king promoted her. In charge of her own battalion, Jeanne's campaigns played a key role in the Dauphin being crowned in 1430. When he was made king, everything seemed to be going The Maiden's way.

Eventually though, Jeanne had been cornered and handed over to the English. In her trial she described how she had "Committed herself to the Lord" and thrown herself off a tower to avoid capture, but those damned Burgundians had turned her over to a pro-English court.

Jeanne was accused of many crimes, but the main one was heresy. The trial had lasted many days. The French King even tried to gain her freedom through ransom, but had failed. He succeeded only in handing over a large sum of money to the English, getting nothing in return.

Today, 30ᵗʰ May 1431, Jeanne was declared guilty of heresy and sentenced to death. This afternoon the 19 year-old girl will be burned at the stake.

The Healer looks one more time at her salve. She wishes she could do more. Her oils seem such a small gesture, but she wants to help the young girl find courage.

The main oil she had chosen was Angelica, grown in a town very close to where Jeanne was to be executed. The plant whose Latin name is Angelica Archangelica helps a person communicate with their angels. It is used in modern times in hospices to help people come to terms with the fact they are about to die.

Many detractors claimed Jeanne was only able to command her army because she drugged them with cannabis, but The Healer has no comment to make on that. She used the herb's cousin, hemp, to relax the girl, Cypress, an oil which fights, protects, and draws strength to your cause, and Dill, an oil that helps young people to ground themselves and fosters common sense.

"Jeanne," whispers The Healer through the prison bars, "Be strong, my girl."

She passes through the pot of oils and holds fervently to the hand which is thrust through. It's so very hard to let go.

As the jailer leads her back through the door, The Healer can longer holdback her tears and wails for the loss of her friend.

Please tell The Healer when you see her....
The verdict of heresy was overturned in 1456. In 1909 Jeanne was beatified by the Vatican, and prayers were made to intercede on her behalf. Blessed, the final part of her journey came in 1920 when she was canonised and declared St Joan. Now she holds the honour of being one of the nine patron saints of France.

Joan of Arc 1412-1431

****

"I'm going to show you Neroli," The Alchemist confides.

Some call it orange blossom, and it's most famous use is for wedding bouquets. In skin care though, it is the elixir of youthful skin for women of more *advanced* years. You watch as he mixes banana, honey, and almonds together to give the skin a vitamin E nourishing feast, and adds his secret ingredient to <u>Ava Gardner's Neroli Mask for Mature Skins</u>.

1963 on the set of <u>7 Days in May</u> with Ava Gardner

The Healer had had enough! Her feet hurt, she had a headache, and if she heard another person shout what number take it was, she may have to use some of the more "suspect" herbs and do the whole lot of them in!

*Gardner might be the face of MGM studios, but she **really** took a long time to make a film. Born in North Carolina, Ava had set her heart on becoming an actress. There was no denying the girl was beautiful... and then some, and boy did it translate onto the screen.*

When The Healer had prepared the girl's skin for her screen test makeup, she had been impressed; translucent, silky smooth, and not an imperfection to be found.

When the MGM screen test came for Al Altman's talent department though, Ava had been shocking! She flubbed her lines, moved awkwardly, and frankly her acting was dreadful. The Healer felt truly sorry for the girl.

However, in the screening room, there was magic afoot. Ava Gardner was mesmerizing, captivating, nothing short of Spectacular!

The Healer would never forget the glee on Altman's face as he leapt from his chair saying, "She can't sing, she can't talk, she can't act...I love it!"

It seemed that from there a star was born.

Starting with a speech coach to obliterate the Southern drawl that no-one could understand, her transformation began.

Ms. Gardner, sits down in her chair, ready for her make up redo... again.

"What can you do to refresh me? I look ...."

"Shhh," says The Healer. "You're just hot. It's nothing a spritz of Neroli can't sort out... orange blossom; quite appropriate really since the film is called 7 days in May! Don't you think?"

With her skin prepared for makeup, the film star returns to the set.

The Healer heads for the sign marked Exit.

Ava Lavinia Gardner 1922-1990

****

Neroli is beautiful, says the alchemist, but let me show you *real* style!

Emeralds, they're not just for anyone you know... it has to be someone *really* special.

You watch as he mixes the carrier oil, which has been charged with the balancing effects of emerald, with drying lavender, and balancing ylang ylang. Then he mashes it into watermelon to give it a cold, hydrating, and cleansing kick. You're being treated to Jackie O's Emerald and Watermelon Mask for Oily Skin.

Natural Beauty

The Healer walks through the door and down the stairs of

Air Force One at 11:45 am on November 22, 1963

The flight to Dallas had been short, and the motorcade had a 9.5 mile trip to the Trade Mart Building where the President was scheduled to make a lunchtime address in his second campaign for office.

The Healer's mistress, Mrs. Kennedy, had had second thoughts about the Pink Chanel suit which The Healer had laid out. She wasn't sure about the hat, but The Healer had reassured her it would be a look that would stay in people's memories for a long time to come; a striking ensemble for a legendary style icon.
On the plane, Jackie had been leafing through magazines looking for inspiration for her renovation of The White House, and trying to distract herself from the loss of her son Patrick, just two days after his birth, three months earlier.

The famous parties in her beautiful home had played a large part in her husband's first election success, but her pregnancy had played more.

In 1960, after a series of difficult pregnancies, doctors had forbidden the soon-to-be First Lady from campaigning with her husband. Instead she stayed home, replied to letters, appeared in TV commercials, and wrote a weekly syndicated newspaper column. Her skills seemed to be endless as she spoke fluently in French and Spanish and even communicated to some voters in Polish and Italian.

Just two weeks after her husband beat Richard Nixon, by a very narrow margin, Jackie gave birth to her first son John F. Kennedy Jr.

In 1961, her husband was inaugurated as the 35th President of the United States, and she became the third youngest First Lady ever.

"Mrs. Kennedy," The Healer hissed as they descended the stairs, "You've left your emerald ring on the table".

"Can you get it for me, please?" she replied, "You can give it to me when we get to the luncheon."

The Healer returned through the airplane door....

Less than an hour later, a gunman shot and killed the President of the United States as he travelled to the luncheon.

Through 1963, Jacqueline Kennedy led her country in mourning for the man who had changed the face of America.

Five years later, she was wed the Greek Shipping magnate Aristotle Onassis, to whom she remained married until his death in '75. The woman born Jacqueline Lee Bouvier, died Jackie Kennedy Onassis in 1994. She is remembered as one of the most important women in American history for her intelligence, strength of character, and her innate sense of style.

Jacqueline Lee Bouvier Kennedy Onassis 1929-1994

****

The Alchemist watches you carefully as you come around. "Do you remember where you were?" He asks carefully. "I was starting to panic, you were away so long. Are you sure you are up to carrying on? That must have been quite a shock."

You take a minute before you steady yourself and say, "OK, let's move along."

The Alchemist is busy mixing a hydrating lotion with rosewater. The rosewater adds hydration but also makes it cooling and nourishing. Rose and geranium oils act like oestrogen for the skin, filling it with rich nurturing goodness. You take a whiff of the Dry Skin Moisturiser and find yourself in

Natural Beauty

Eleanor Roosevelt's Rose Garden at Springwood Estate, Hyde Park, NY

The Healer walks slowly through the garden and lays a yellow rose on the grave of the great Eleanor Roosevelt.

Her heart feels heavy for the country's loss. Mind you, 78 was a ripe old age, and The Healer's old friend had, had a good run.

Born Anna Eleanor Roosevelt in 1884, her parents had both died when she was a young girl. At school, she was tutored by a feminist headmistress who was to play a part in the restructuring of America's rights for women.

In 1905, Eleanor married her fifth cousin Franklin D. Roosevelt, but from the beginning, their marriage was hard. A meddling mother-in-law and a dalliance on his part persuaded Eleanor to search for more independence.

She encouraged Franklin to continue his interest in politics and often took the place of her husband, partially paralysed by polio, at speeches and rallies.

She had often been outspoken, and The Healer wondered how her friend had ever dared oppose her husband's policies so openly. She campaigned for rights of women in the workplace, for civil rights of African Americans and Asian Americans, and for WWII refugees.

Twelve years was a long time to live in The White House.

After her husband's death in 1945, Eleanor had continued in politics, and, at the end of her life, had even served as part of the JFK administration working for women's rights.

At the time of her death, she was considered to be one of the most esteemed women in the world.

The yellow rose had been her friend's favourite, and now the flower, so helpful in the treatment of grief, seemed to be an appropriate token.

A memory made The Healer smile, the longest-serving First Lady in history had been quite put out with the catalogue's description of the rose which bore her name, "No good in a bed, but fine up against a wall!"

Buffeted by mirth...The Healer walked through the front door of the house and disappeared.

Eleanor Roosevelt 1884-1962

On your return, the alchemist wants to know if you are ready to see something really remarkable.

You can't quite imagine how anything could be more amazing than what you have already seen, but you watch as he collects his ingredients. Nothing could have prepared you for the sights and smells you were about to witness.

He blends aloe vera, which is cooling and gentle, with nurturing rose quartz, relaxing camomile, violet, and palmarosa, which are gentle to both the skin and the spirit, to concoct <u>Mother Theresa' Rose Quartz Tranquillity Mask</u>

The Streets of Calcutta

The Healer is worried as she walks through the door into this filthy street. Flies circle around her, and the stench of infection fills the air. It is a breezeless, scorching day. All around is decay; people with rotting skin, and sores, struggling for breath. In these desperate surroundings there is, however, a strange sense of hope. The Healer thinks the nun should be resting, but alas, Theresa will not be told. For many months now the nun has been ailing, but today she is insistent – she must see her friend.

Natural Beauty

The Princess of Wales visits today away from the glare of the paparazzi flash bulbs. Unbeknownst to the rest of the world, the kindred spirits will walk the streets of Calcutta in privacy.

The two women have been friends since the Princess flew to Rome to meet the nun in 1992. The princess had wanted to see the work amongst the squalor for herself, but she knew the media would become a circus. The Healer had come up with the plan for them to walk the back streets and secretly visit alone. Now when she saw how frail her dear friend Mother Theresa had become, she wondered whether her plan had been wise.

Mother Theresa had been born in 1910 to Albanian parents and baptised Anjeze Gonxhe Bojahiu meaning Little Rose Bud or Tiny Flower.

The nun took her orders in 1937 and had been living by what she called "her vows" ever since: three of the convent: Chastity, Poverty, Obedience, and to those she added, whole-hearted service to the poorest of the poor.

To those vows, she had been true. Creating hospices for HIV/AIDs, Tuberculosis, even leprosy. The Healer rolled her eyes when she thought of the criticism the nun received for the state of her hospices. What would those people have if the hospices closed? As for complaining about her campaigns against contraception... which part of "Catholic Nun," didn't they get?!

The two women greeted The Healer warmly as Mother Theresa held out her hand.

"Thank you," she said. "It helps centre my compassion," she explained as she showed the pink stone.

Diana nodded and smiled wryly to The Healer "You don't have any rosewater with you, do you?"

It was a long, hot day before The Healer left through a humble shack door that evening.

When you see The Healer, please can you tell her...

I'm sorry for her loss. Two incredible spirits were taken in the summer of 1997 just six days apart. The earth became a poorer place without them both.

Mother Theresa's legacy continues on. In 2012, The Missionaries of Charity had over 4500 sisters in 133 countries running hospices, soup kitchen and clinics.

Mother Theresa 1910-1997

****

"You look hot" said the alchemist. Let me show you how to make another type of toner to cool you down.
He mixes rose, rose, and more rose in <u>Princess Diana's Rosewater Toner</u> for a megablast of cooling nourishment.

July 29, 1981 Princess Diana's Wedding Carriage

The Healer looked around, thinking, "That was a first!"

She'd just come out of the door of a carriage. That was pretty cool, but it also meant rather than sneaking in and out of historic scenes discretely as she was supposed to, it was possible 750 million TV viewers around the world had just seen her "materialize."

Note to self... work on "entrances!"

In front of her lay miles of ivory silk. It was the wedding gown of Lady Diana Spencer, soon to be the Princess of Wales.

The young nursery school teacher had had a lot to learn when she was first introduced to The Healer, not the least of which was about the press. The poor girl had been mortified when the papers had printed the picture of her with the sun shining through her skirt, even though she certainly had a cracking pair of legs on her.

Over the ensuing months, The Healer had not left her side, always with the same small bottle at hand.

"Rosewater to cool a princess..." that's what she had said. Cooling and centring, there was no other plant that could make a woman feel quite so feminine.

After her obligatory quick spray, the Princess had heaved her enormous Emmanuel dress out of the carriage, and glided up to St Paul's Cathedral.

Normally The Healer would have left the scene a bit earlier, but didn't everyone want to see this Royal Wedding? A quick sneak peek wouldn't do any harm.

She found a quiet spot at the back of the cathedral as the Jeremiah Clark's Trumpet Voluntary bounced around the walls.

The Healer could not help but wonder if this enigmatic and beautiful girl was made of strong enough stuff for all of this.

Wiping a tear of joy from her eye, she left St Paul's.

When you see The Healer please will you tell her...

The Princess went on to give birth to two sons who were to be second and third in line to the throne, until the Princess's first grandson was born in 2013, taking the third place spot. The pressures of the press played a large part in her tragic long-term fight with eating disorders. The world came to love her compassionate spirit and soft demeanour. In 1996 her marriage to Prince Charles ended when they divorced after numerous stories of their respective love affairs.

On August 31, 1997, The Healer's fears came true when Diana and her companion, Dodi Al Fayed, were killed in a car crash in Paris while racing away from paparazzi. Or that's what they'd have us believe any way....

Diana, Princess of Wales 1961-1997

****

The Alchemist has nothing snarky to comment as you return, he merely says he wants to show you how to make <u>Elizabeth I's Nourishing Agarwood Acne Moisturiser</u>. You watch as he creates a blend of agarwood and jasmine to alleviate the scarring, and sandalwood to reduce the heat and to kill any infection.

When it is complete, you inhale deeply. The rich and heady exotics soon tempt you back in time.

Through the door, The Healer can hear the frenzy of the crowd which awaits her. As she fights her way through to the palace...

1562 The court of Queen Elizabeth I

What more could life throw at Elizabeth, wondered The Healer? Actually, it didn't bear thinking about, so perhaps she didn't want to know.

The princess Elizabeth had been born to Henry VIII and his second wife Anne Boleyn. Her mother was beheaded when the young Elizabeth was just two and a half years old, and the child was declared illegitimate and stripped of her place in the line to the throne. Despite this, Elizabeth worked hard to become the most educated woman of her generation, speaking nine languages fluently by the time of her death.

At age 14, after the death of her father King Henry, she was taken into the home of her stepmother Catherine Parr. Parr's new husband had pursued and sexually abused the young Elizabeth. Perhaps this had contributed to her lack of an heir, The Healer mused. What was certain, was Elizabeth was not the "Virgin Queen" people liked to claim she was.

The Healer could think of many a wife who might have a gripe with their husband's regal dalliances!

Elizabeth had watched patiently from the wings as her brother Edward, Lady Jayne Grey, and finally her sister Mary had all taken the throne and perished.

Now three years after Elizabeth's own coronation, the queen had contracted small pox. The Healer had bought a salve to try to calm the effects of the disease. The agarwood would treat the small pox, and the jasmine was chosen to heal her scars. The tea tree and lemon were chosen to fight the infection and geranium to generate healthy cells, The Healer wanted so much to help her beautiful strong queen.

Passing the salve to the guard in front of the bedchamber, The Healer fought her way back through the crowds.

When you see The Healer please tell her....

Elizabeth I is fondly remembered for what is termed The Golden Age of England. Drama and the arts flourished, thanks to Shakespeare and Marlow. Francis Drake and his privateers saw to it that the country benefited greatly from his exploration of the seas and plundering of ports. She ruled the country defensively, regularly swapping allegiances with France and Spain. Spain finally pushed her too far, and the Armada was destroyed, bringing Elizabeth one of the greatest military victories the country has ever enjoyed.

Sadly though, the guard never passed on The Healer's salve, and Elizabeth's skin became hideously disfigured by small pox scars. By the end of her life, she was no longer the beauty The Healer would have remembered.

Elizabeth I of England, 1533-1603

****

The alchemist just sighs a rueful smiles and says, "A moisturiser for a mature lady's skin then?"

He mixes a hydrating lotion with the rich skin healer calendula, adds orange and tangerine to refine the skin and close the pores, and benzoin to encourage new, fresh cell growth. You lean in for a sniff as he pronounces <u>Salome's Moisturiser for Mature Skins</u> complete.

As The Healer approaches the door, she is spitting with rage. She cannot believe the little girl she saw grow up could have turned into such a spiteful little cat! The cream was allegedly to moisturise the girl's skin after her bath, but really, it had a more subtle lesson for the girl to learn. The Healer supposed it had a lot to do with the mother. Strange morals, that one had, that's for sure. Clutching the pot of cream, The Healer stormed into

AD 33 The bedroom of Salome

Salome was the daughter of Herod II and Herodias. She was a spoiled creature at the best of times, but this time she had really gone too far.

As The Healer approached the room, she averted her eyes to prevent her from looking at the grotesque head which stared up from the plate.

John the Baptist had spoken out and angered her mother Herodias, by declaring Herodias' new marriage to Herod Antipas unlawful. Salome's mother had previously been married to Herod Antipas' half-brother, Salome's father (Herod II), and then had divorced him.

Whether the Baptist had been right or not in his opinions, voicing them had been a fatal mistake.

Herodias' daughter was famous for her exotic dancing, which delighted anyone who watched. Last week, Salome's father had asked her to entertain his palace guests with her talent. So graceful and tempting was she, Herod summoned her to him, proudly declaring he would grant his daughter any wish she desired. He even offered her half his kingdom, but Salome was not to be persuaded.

She ordered the Baptist's head to be delivered to her on a silver platter.

Herod, angst-ridden by her request, had begged her to change her mind, knowing the execution to be wrong, but the spoiled little miss was resolute, and the king had made a promise.

The Healer smashed the cream down beside Salome's bath and walked away. She was simply too angry to speak to the girl. The rich body cream she had made was filled with oils which The Healer hoped would one day make Salome understand what she had done; orange oil to encourage her to see what she is capable of, Calendula, an oil which helps people in authority make good decisions, and benzoin to help her understand moral concepts.

The Healer stomped back through the door and slammed it closed behind her.

Salome AD 14-31

****

The Alchemist shows you a bowl of exotic looking ingredients. It is an all-over exfoliating rub he explains. You know now how blissful these treatments are, and you lie back as he applies Scheherazade's Exfoliating Rub and wait for The Healer to return.

He mixes nurturing rose, geranium, and sandalwood, with regenerating lemon, into a rich, nourishing, and refreshing coconut oil.

The Persian Legend of Sheherezade

The Healer skips along the corridor, eager to see the triumph of the girl whom she loves so dearly. Unlike the others whom The Healer has watched seduce through their beauty and grace, this clever thing uses wiles and wisdom to bag her man. Her charm is born through learning, study, and imagination. The Healer wishes more girls looked to this women as a role-model.

The beguiling Scheherzade, daughter of the great Vizier serving in the court of King Sharbriya, seemed to have their rather unusual ruler eating out of her hand.

The Healer LOVED it! Clever, clever, girl....

*Things had been more than slightly strained since the King had lost his first wife. Lost... is perhaps **not** the best word to use, but it seems kinder somehow. He had been desperately in love with the woman, but she had betrayed him.*

In anger, he killed her and took a new wife, then another, and another. For 1000 days he found a virgin, married her, and then beheaded her the next day, marrying her successor.

Like I say.... a little "strained."

The Healer chuckled to herself as she mused that young Sheherezade is not your traditional beauty heroine.

As a child she had been a bit of a bookworm, really. She had read books about great rulers and their military campaigns, and she could recite poetry. Her encyclopaedic knowledge was coupled with a fertile imagination and a most charismatic way with words.

The Healer could not imagine the father's horror when one day his little scholar volunteered herself as a virgin for the king. That poor man! Deaf to her father's pleas, Sheherezade put herself forward and was duly chosen as bride.

Natural Beauty

The Healer was glad the girl had confided her plan and asked her for her help.

On the night of the wedding, Scheherazade had asked the king for the favour of saying one last goodbye to her beloved sister, which he granted. The wily Dinazade, already primed by her sister, played her part magnificently, and asked Scheherezade to tell her "just one more story."

So she did.

The most romantic, evocative, mesmerising, thrilling, and hypnotic tale she could muster tripped lightly from the brides' mouth. For hours the king listened, beguiled. Then suddenly she stopped, apologising for being too tired to continue. Despite being begged by the king to tell him how it ended, the enchantress refused, and won herself a stay of execution of one more day.

The next evening she continued the story and began a new one, which of course was not concluded... until the following evening.

And now, The Healer entered with her blend of lemon and flowers as she had made every night. Scheherezade would massage her legs seductively with the mix as she cast yet another spell. The lemon and roses would aid her story telling and creative spirit.

Reassured now, that the young virgin knew precisely what she was doing, The Healer laid the pot of oils onto the opulent bed covers and left the room.

When you see The Healer, please will you tell her...

Through 1001 nights, Sheherezade narrated her way to another day, until finally the King realized what every girl could have guessed from day one. He had fallen in love. Sheherezade was made his queen, and they all lived happily ever after.

****

As you come to, The Alchemist is chuckling... "Wasn't she great?" You start to say how fascinating Scheherazade must have been, but he simply puts a finger to his lips and shakes his head, and starts to explain how the next treatment will detoxify and cleanse your body.

He prepares a blend of homemade dandelion infusion, with Inula, fennel, and cypress to flush toxins out of the body, then combines it with green clay. The clay cleanses so deeply, with its diuretic effects, that <u>Helen of Troy's Hell-in-A Pair of Skinny Jeans</u> will usually shave between a half and a whole inch off your hips and thighs!

With the slightly strange sensation of clay drying and caking over your skin, a now familiar journey begins again.

The Palace Gardens with Helen in Troy

The Healer likes it when she gets to go to the time of Greek Gods and Mount Olympus, full of handsome men and mythical beasts! She is visiting Helen of Sparta, the daughter of Zeus and Leda, and sister of Castor Pollux and Clytemnestra. Helen, considered to be the most beautiful woman in the word, was abducted by Paris, thus sparking the Trojan War. Ever heard the saying, "The Face that Launched a Thousand Ships?" That was Helen.

Distraught at the chaos she had caused, Helen was inconsolable. The Healer felt she needed to give the girl a bit of support and calm her down.

Helen would not be coaxed with a cup of tea, so The Healer suggested a walk in the garden. As Helen began to weep, her tears fell to the ground. The Healer watched in disbelief as Elecampane, an orange daisy-like flower with a bittersweet scent, sprang from the dampened soil.

The Healer often used the essential oil from this plant, known as Inula (its Latin name is Inula helenium) to heal respiratory complaints, but it was also very effective for bloating and menstrual problems.

Useful, you thought, as you devised a plan to see how the plant might deal with water retention.

When Helen seemed to be a little calmer, you rushed back to the temple to try out your new idea.

****

As you come back to the Spa, there's something tickling in the back of your mind. You turn to The Alchemist and exclaim, "Wait a minute, *I* created Hell-in-a Pair of Skinny Jeans, didn't I?!?"

The Alchemist smiles wryly. "Yes my dear, I see the tea and treatments have finally done their work. These are all your ideas, all your experiences. You have helped a great many people in your incarnations. It's my place to merely help you remember that *you* are The Healer. You can now use your unlocked knowledge to create whatever you need to enhance your own beauty and that of others, and to heal on many levels. In just a bit, I'm going to share a couple of my own creations with you as well, but before we do that... a few final bits of skin care... before we adorn you. Do you remember this one?"

At the herb cupboard he collects the ingredients for <u>Shea Butter with Jasmine, Patchouli, and Neroli</u>. He mixes together the richest, sexiest, and utterly wonderful oils with the silky opulence of shea. This is a nourishing and tantalising cream....and then some!

1370 BC The City of Luxor with Queen Nefertiti

Here, The Healer is very young in her incarnations. She is proud to be an apprentice of the bedchamber for the queen of the Egyptians, Nefertiti who, by the way, was to become one of the most celebrated women of ancient civilisation.

The apprentice healer loves learning from her queen. She adores her new home in the majestic city of Luxor. Most of all, she relishes the view from her window overlooking the Nile valley lush with its palm trees.

Nefertiti, and her husband the great Pharaoh Akhenaten, had revolutionized Egypt in every way imaginable. The country was rich and the economy had never been so strong. Their capital city had moved to Luxor and her master and mistress had even overhauled the entire religious expression of the civilisation, turning their praises from their many gods to the monotheistic religion of the Great Aten.

Never had the great civilisation had it so good.

Recently though, Akenaten had died. Now Nefertiti ruled the country, for a short while anyway, in readiness for her son to take the throne when he eventually came of age.

The young healer watched as the queen showed her how to break the shea nuts and grind them to make a cream. She smiled shyly as Nefertiti said, "Who knows, you might even be able to make healing creams yourself one day."

As you return from your adventure in Egypt you recall......

Three thousand years later, Nefertiti's boy king become the face which would become synonymous with Egyptian culture, Tutankamen.

Nefertiti was a strong and revered ruler, much loved by her people. Because she was so well depicted in illustration and sculpture of the time, we understand why the queen's beauty was so admired.

Natural Beauty

In the British museum is a near perfect bust which shows her angular features and regal brow. Hieroglyphics depict the queen beautifying herself with what historians suspect could be Shea Butter.

Nefertiti circa 1370 -1340BC

****

And finally says the alchemist, let's have a look at those feet!

He mixes the cooling and anti-bacterial ingredients of spikenard, sandalwood, and lavender with ice cold peppermint and relaxing camomile and yarrow to create <u>Mary Magdalene's Foot Balm of Biblical Proportions.</u>

Mary Magdalene in the Home of Lazarus in Bethany

When The Healer enters the little house in Bethany, the atmosphere is electric. Mary, the sister of Lazarus had invited The Teacher to her home. The man they called Jesus was holding court, and everyone seemed so excited to have him there.

No wonder, the man was a bit of a hero. Mary, especially, thought so, since she was convinced her brother had been dead, and yet this Jesus had raised him up. Mary felt she owed him everything.

The other Mary, the one they called Magdalene, watched quietly in the corner. The Healer wished she could work that one out. Some said she was a woman of ill repute, but she had never seen anything to point to that. Still, perhaps there was no smoke without fire.

The previous week the Magdalene had asked The Healer if she could acquire some Nard. So naturally The Healer had agreed. Lazarus's sister had washed the Teacher's feet with the oil before to refresh them.

The Healer wondered if Magdalene would do the same and gave her the oil.

Shaking your head you remember.....

In the book we call The Bible, a woman, a penitent sinner, washes Jesus's feet. We do not know whether it was Mary Magdalene, or even if the job description of "ill repute" did in fact fit.

Nevertheless, the church labelled her, whore. In 1969, they retracted the reference, saying there was no evidence she was the penitent sinner. Of course, the connection still lingers.

Theories today abound as to whether she and Jesus eventually married. Some say a holy blood line was born from her, and you like that idea, but we will probably never know.

****

The Alchemist seems very happy with how things are going, as he strokes your skin and nods approvingly.

Now we are ready for a bit of decoration, he says.

He mixes and applies <u>Boudicca's War Paint</u>!

The Healer walks through the door into a classroom full of twentieth century beauty students. "Let me tell you about a woman I once knew who liked to wear woad"

AD 60 Boudica in Roman Britain

The flame-haired warrior queen of the Iceni battled against the Romans from East Anglia to North Wales. When the Romans invaded England in AD43, they allowed her husband Prasutagus to continue to rule, but on his death, they confiscated the lands of the major landowners and decided to rule themselves.

Incandescent with rage, his widow rose up and led an army of men right across Albion. Adorned with their traditional war paint, they must have looked a fearsome battalion. Their frenzied red hair trailing behind then, lips stained red with blackberry juice, bright against their milky white skins, fingernails stained blood red with elder juice, and frenzied blue artistry scrawled over their faces. The bright lapis blue was made from a native herb of the area, woad. As they screamed over the hills with their cudgels and lances, I am sure the Romans thought twice about advancing.

Boudicca's army successfully overthrew the mighty ninth legion and rallied by their victory, headed on to take the capital of Roman Britain, Colchester. Onward, they took London and then St. Albans. The bloodshed was terrifying. Thousands of Britons died. Boudicca was finally defeated, and it is thought she may have poisoned herself to deny the Romans the pleasure of her capture.

Now feel free to try this with woad, which would have been blended with stale urine, back in the day. These days if you want to use it as an eyeliner or eye shadow, the bright, vibrant colour has absolutely no synthetic comparison. Mix it with alcohol to a runny paste and then paint on.

But I have a far more <u>glamorous option</u>, The Alchemist taught me this...

Boudica – Birthdate unknown. Died AD 60

****

Now, says the alchemist, I'm going to dust your body with powdered pearls. Not only does it shimmer beautifully, but it will soothe your nerves and instil confidence.

He takes a large powder brush and applies <u>Marilyn Monroe's Powder Blush.</u>

1960 the Dressing Room of Marilyn Monroe

As The Healer pushes the door to the studio open with her hip, she can hear the director swearing. Where is she? What's the crisis this time? The Healer knows then that Marilyn didn't make it to work. She picks up the phone to call the screen icon.

There's no reply, but in her dressing room The Healer notices the 16" strand of pearls that Jo DiMaggio gave her lies discarded on the table. She picks them up and heads over to the film star's room.

She knocks, and an attendant lets her in. The beautiful Monroe is sobbing, nervous as usual about her takes. The Healer sits down beside her as the fragile film star's words tumble out in streams of almost incoherent babble about not good enough, can't do it, failure.

Gently The Healer picks up the pearls and places them around her milky white throat.

The energy of the beads soothes her. As the mood slowly lifts, the actress begins to see what the rest of the world sees.

Washing her face and putting on her makeup, Marilyn Monroe returns to the set.

Norma Jean Mortensen 1926-62

****

You look radiant, says the alchemist. I have one last gift to give you before you go.
You can take this one home with you. It's gift that should be shared with someone special…

Natural Beauty

You inhale the rich cocoa of the <u>Edible Body Chocolate</u> <u>Flecked with Gold.</u> It's invigorating and stimulating, especially with the added hit of caffeine, and the vanilla that is an aphrodisiac too.

You look at The Alchemist, and he just winks and flashes those pearly whites again...

As you're leaving the room, you have the odd sense of being watched.

You walk through the door and for just a moment, imagine you see a figure beside you. No, you think, it must be a trick of the light... nothing more than a shadow.

And yet you could have sworn you saw The Healer...

What strange things we learn in the quietness of "me time"

Could it be perhaps, you just "remembered" a healer's knowledge?

Part 2

Beauty Through the Ages

From the moment our biology first experienced attraction, there has been a physiological need to try to enhance that which we have. For eons, people have been using plants, precious metals, and oils to make the very best of what they have got.

The process of attraction was complex, however, because relationships were never only between two people, but always included their families, countries, and their gods. In many civilisations, great rituals were performed with magical essences in the hope to tempt their deities a little closer.

When the tomb of Tutankhamen was opened, archaeologists found tears of frankincense and myrrh. We know these were used in the mummification rituals, but also in their communications with gods.

The cosmetics we wear today take their influences from the khol worn by the pharaohs. Though it may be tempting to imagine that Egypt birthed many of these traditions, the truth is it seems that way simply because that is where the bulk of the existing evidence lies.

What Is Beauty Anyway?

I suppose I should open this section with a disclaimer. Not every woman whom I deem to be unforgettable made the cut. Yoko Ono, Charlotte Brontë, and Sarah Bernhardt, for instance, were on the original list. Helen Keller, Marie Curie, and Princess Grace inspired me too.

Natural Beauty

The problem is of course, memorable is simple to define, but beauty, not so much.

More complicated still, one person's perception of what is aesthetically pleasing may be shockingly different from your own. Thank goodness for that too, as this is one of the things which guarantees we continue to procreate! However, it does make for difficult choices for a book.

Scientists come up with a million different ideas of what might make the perfect face, symmetry, biology, and of course plastic surgery, but in the end I think we would all agree...

Beauty is some kind of fire behind the eyes. A purpose, a confidence, and an assurance in a person makes them far more attractive to anyone looking on.

For these are our leaders, our thinkers, and the ones whom we choose to follow to change how our world works; therefore their stories survive in their wake.

Beauty From a Holistic Point of View

Holistic healing takes its beauty dimension from Ayurveda, which is often thought of as the Mother of Medicines. It considers beauty in a very different way than our more contemporary ideals of stick-thin models who pout at us from magazine covers.

The holistic healing model fits very well into the principle of the mind, the body, and the spirit of the naturally beautiful woman. Rather than only addressing the bone structure, complexion, and hip ratio of the creature, holistic beauty looks at the face as only one aspect of her appeal.

In fact, we look at it in terms of three: the outer body, the inner body, and also the secret aspect of the girl (or boy! Ayurveda makes no distinction).

The outer body is what is perceived by the outside world, skin, bone structure, hair, nails, and teeth.

To the inner body, apart from the obvious digestive processes and what might leave the body, we would also include thoughts, and internal processing in general.

When the inner body and the outer body work well together, the secret aspect seems to shine from the woman like the most radiant jewel.

Given this then, when the body and mind are nourished in a way that engages and galvanises a woman, her appeal is increased one hundred fold. Many of the women in our little jaunt through time were classically beautiful, but *all* are memorable; their incredible sense of purpose, their joy, and even when they plunged into despair in order to fulfil their destinies. These women are the stuff of legend, which for many of us seems entirely removed from our own realities.

Any yet, we have around us just the same qualities and exactly the same tools at our disposal to create our own individual place of both greatness and serenity.

Our Unforgettable Women had plants, they had gems and soils, and they had herbs. So do we. In our world of interconnectedness, we should be able to build brighter, stronger, more energetic futures than ever they did but where on earth do we start?

Look in the mirror, Snow White… it has something to tell you…..

Key Components of a Beauty Regime

For any of the skin on your body to gleam with health, whether it is your facial complexion or your flabbier thighs, there are four vital components...
1. Cleansing
2. Exfoliating
3. Moisturising
4. Nourishing

To understand how these work, it helps to have a cursory knowledge of how the skin works.

The Skin
It is the largest organ in the body and it has several functions.

1. It keeps water inside the body.
2. It keeps bacteria out.
3. It protects the internal organs.
4. It houses the hair follicles and sebaceous glands which produce vital anti-bacterial agents.
5. It regulates temperature.

The skin is made up of three layers.

Epidermis
The skin which you see on the surface is made up entirely of dead skin cells. These are made up of a hard protein called keratin, which also makes up the structure of hair and nails. This surface is constantly shedding cells. We recognise this as dust in the air sometimes.

In some parts of the body this layer of cells is thin. We call this epithelial tissue. A good example of this is where you can see good blood supply beneath the surface, e.g., the lips and the insides of the wrist.

Compound epithelial tissue is strong and course and sheds with more difficulty. For an example of this, consider the heels of your feet.

The Dermis
Here, the skin cells mature and develop proteins. These cells are called keratinocytes. When their life cycle is complete they are pushed up through to the epidermis.

Granular Layer
Sometimes you may also see this referred to as the basal layer. It is richly supplied with capillaries which form the connection with the subcutaneous layer. This is where new skin cells are made. They are then pushed up to the dermis.

You may also be familiar with the effect of goose bumps on the skin when muscles called the erector pilli signal changes in temperature or perhaps of excitement of fear. These are left over from a days of Neanderthal man, when our bodies would have been completely covered in hair. On the surface, they may seem to be now redundant. However in each follicle exists a sebaceous gland. These secrete sebum, an oily substance which cleanses the skin of bacteria. Problems happen when the sebaceous glands decide to secrete too little, making the skin dry and flaky, or over produce creating that oil slick complexion we had as teenagers. This of course means greasy skin can happen at any age to anyone.

The very base of the skin is made up of subcutaneous fat. You will recognise how the plumpness of this can make people look younger. Its function is to keep us warm. If you look at the faces of the Eskimo peoples, you will see they have formed very thick lids to protect their eyes.

Caring for the Skin

Cleansing
This involves ridding the skin of any debris which maybe causing it harm. It may mean treating black heads or even pollution you have absorbed from the air.

You will remember the sebaceous glands and their oily substance, sebum. Regularly cleaning this off the skin helps it to produce more normally and healthily.

Exfoliation
Once you understand how the skin is made, it helps you to see why exfoliation is very useful. By sloughing off the outer dead skin cells, it forces new younger-looking ones to the surface. This gives the skin a youthful translucency. It also encourages blood flow in the skin.

Above all other things, exfoliation is the key to beautiful skin.

Moisturising
All skin needs moisturising. It may seem counter intuitive to say that about greasy skin, but the clue is in the name. Many creams you put on your skin are made from waxes and heavy oils. All this does is coat the skin and trick the sebaceous glands into performing even more badly.

Moisturising is done with a water based cream. In this book I use a blend of nourishing beeswax and herbal tea to make the base of the treatment. It drenches the skin with water and your skin will love you for it.

At this point I will also say drink more water too. Since the skin does not need water for any vital process, the body starves it to conserve more for the rest of the body. If you have dry skin, the first step in sorting it out is to up your fluid intake.

Nourishing

For the most part, this is where the essential oils and plants come in. Think of it as food for your skin. A great example is the potted plants on your patio. If you don't feed them, they start to loose vitality as they use up all their composted resources. The skin works in exactly the same way. Nourishing them with essential oils and crystal elixirs can improve the skin overnight.

Natural Ingredients for Beautiful Creatures

Essential oils

This book is focused mainly (but not exclusively) around essential oils, the concentrated essences of plants. They are nothing short of miraculous, in that they are able to absorb through the skin and into the blood system. Once there, they are able to manipulate the hormones in our bodies to align them to health. So for example, we use lavender oil for greasy skin, as it balances sebum production.

For the purpose of this book, I shall focus mainly on beauty oils, but of course they can heal in a million different ways. You might also want to read *Nature's Medicine*, where I explore how to heal more common ailments using oils and herbs.

Holistic treatments differ from more traditional approaches in that they treat the individual as a person, rather than just their symptoms.

The recipes at the end of the book depend on the fact that essential oils do not have side effects, but instead, many main effects. Let me repeat that, "essential oils do not have *side* effects, but instead, many *main* effects." This idea is fundamental to the book.

As well as physical effects, an oil will usually have emotional and mental effects too. Taking lavender as an example, we know it balances sebum, but it is also relaxing, soothing, antiviral, and it helps burns. You will start to understand this better as this section unfolds.

Essential oils are extremely potent, and so should be diluted into some type of base, whether it be a carrier oil, or a cream, or a lotion. They can also be used in the bath.

The main oils which we use for skin care are:

Agarwood -Aquilaria malaccensis
This is one of the most expensive oils found anywhere in the world, costing around $13,000 an ounce for the really good stuff. More affordable versions can be had with a sixteenth of an ounce costing a little less than $50! It is extremely aphrodisiac, is cooling for hot and sore skin, and is deeply relaxing. It calms anxiety and opens up cerebral processing.

Other uses:
Medicinally, it is used to treat both respiratory and digestive problems.

Angelica Root- Angelica archangelica
The angelica plant is tall and statuesque. Its roots reach deep into the earth to keep it erect. These roots are thirsty creatures and suck up any moisture they can find. When the essential oil is used on the body, it gushes all that glorious hydration back into the skin.

In beauty treatments, it softens and reenergises lacklustre complexions, and it takes away redness and whitens the skin.

Other uses:
Digestive complaints

Bergamot – Citrus Bergamia
This is a kind of green orange that grows in the city of Bergamo in southern Italy.
It is a very uplifting oil. It smells like a cross between an orange and a lime, which is exactly what it is.

Bergamot is an extremely good cleanser. It cuts through the grime on your complexion. It is also a lovely, invigorating oil which stimulates the circulation beneath the surface and bring a lovely fresh glow to the skin. It also will reduce breakouts of acne.

Other uses:
Bergamot is sunshine in a bottle. It is used for depression, for uplifting the spirits, and also has an effect on reducing your weight.

Camomile - Camomile Maroc
I love everything about camomile. In fact, I have planted a camomile lawn in my garden so I can bliss out when I am not working. The oils are released as I tread on the soft green carpet.

It is called the earth apple, and its scent is indeed reminiscent of the fruit. In fact, there are three different types of camomile oil which we use in therapy, but for a beginner I would recommend you get some *camomile maroc.*

It is very soothing, so if the skin is hot and red, not only will it cool it, but it will also reduce the redness. It is anti–inflammatory, so it reduces puffiness and swelling which is useful for "morning after eyes," for example.

The other oils do pretty much the same, but in stronger capacity. Camomile roman smells very similar to maroc, but is more anti-inflammatory. Camomile matricaria is just a little bit special, but you'll pay for it. It is a deep, rich, blue oil, due to a constituent called Azulene, which is like liquid anaesthetic. The other oil you will see this in is spikenard. Both of them are emergency helpers when there is excruciating pain or upset.

Other uses:

If it's swollen, if it hurts, if it is upset (you can say this for stomach for instance, or mood) then get your camomile out of your box.

Carrot – Daucus Carota

Carrot is such an important oil for cleaning pollution off the skin. All the debris in the air, cigarette smoke, and smog, which toughen the skin, and even grimy sebum.

It is a must-have oil for great skin.

Other uses
It is very good for digestive complaints, especially flatulence (pardon me!), and it is also a tonic for the liver.

Cypress – Cypressus Semperivens

Cypress, cypress how I love thee.

I sit in front of a computer screen most days, and so my skin is constantly exposed to the effects of positive ions which not only toughen the skin and make it look grey, but also can open you up to headaches, dizziness, and a fuzzy head.

Grab your bottle of cypress, and it will also reduce bloating and swelling in the face too, since it has lymphatic properties.

Other uses:
Menstrual problems are aided as it regulates blood flow, and it also relaxes muscles.

Frankincense - Boswellia Carterii

Yes, this is the same oil which was brought by the magi for the Christ child. At the time, it would have been far more valuable than the gold and would most likely have been in its incense form. The incense is collected by slashing a cut into the bark of a tree and then letting the resin drip out.

When the resin is dry, fragments are broken off. These are called "tears."

The Egyptians used frankincense to embalm their mummies, which shows just how good a preservation material it is. Frankincense is for the most mature of skins.

Other uses:
It preserves by holding onto elasticity. This is also very helpful if you need to treat a strained tendon. It is used for respiratory complaints, is a decongestant, and it helps to slow down the breath. For this reason, it is also aligned with prayer and meditation and is burned in the high churches.

Emotionally, frankincense is wonderful for instilling confidence.

Geranium – Pelargonium Graveolens
Some books suggest to use geranium if you cannot afford to get any rose. This implies that it is an inferior choice, but in fact geranium is a healing star in its own right.

Yes, it is nourishing like rose, and affects the hormones, but it also invigorates circulation and supports the adrenals.

Other uses:
When the world has given you a bit of a kicking, I recommend you lie in a bath of geranium. The day just melts away. Geranium is also very soothing for feeding mothers whose breasts have become compacted and sore.
Emotionally, geranium is very calming. Imagine the way a cup of tea helps to put things into perspective. Geranium does the same.

Grapefruit – Citrus Paradisii
Anyone who has been on a diet probably knows grapefruit helps to break down fat. It's true, it does. It works on the

liver to help the body metabolise fat. In this way, it helps with weight loss and with cellulite in particular. It is extremely astringent and cleansing to the skin. It is amazing for blackheads. It is also very good for improving the lymphatic system.

Other uses
It is very refreshing to the spirit. Use it also to help colds and flu because of its high content of vitamin C.

Jasmine – Jasminum Officinalis
The heady scent of jasmine is bottled to make the oil of the flower called the King of the flowers. Who can blame them? Where rose is the most effective oil for healing gynaecological problems, jasmine is the male equivalent, but any girl who turns her back on the rich sensuous oil is missing a trick.

It is incredible for soothing hot and sore skins, so think acne and rosacea for example.

Other uses:
It is a tonic for the womb, which means pregnant women are advised to avoid until labour has begun. It is highly aphrodisiac by releasing inhibitions and stress. It is an all over tonic to the reproductive system. If you say sex, you mean jasmine.

Lavender - Lavendula Angustifola
Lavender is the go-to oil in aromatherapy, but many people don't realise they may be inadvertently creating skin care problems for themselves by using it. Lavender oil is actually for greasy skin. The reason we choose it is because it communicates with the sebaceous glands which make oils for the skin, and instructs them to reduce production.

Relax in lavender oil baths for too long, you will soon notice dryness appearing.

Other uses:
Everything in the world…and then some. Most notably, it is wonderful for treating burns. It is relaxing and soothing. It is antibacterial and anti-biotic. It brings wonderful pain relief, of both the physical and emotional sorts.

Melissa - Melissa Officinalis
Springtime in a bottle! Melissa is used in skin care for two reasons. Number one, it is astringent, so it makes a lovely refreshing choice for a toner. Secondly, it reduces allergies, many of which can be the trigger for sensitive skins.

Other uses: The most emotionally uplifting of all the oils. It can help any kind of allergy, in particular, hay fever.

Myrrh - Myrrhus Communis
Myrrh is a skin healer, rather than a skin *care* oil. By that I mean, abscesses, cuts, abrasions, grazes are all healed by myrrh. It has the effect of knitting the skin of even deep fissures.

Other uses:
It is has antibiotic properties and so cleanses wounds of bacteria. It is a very sedative oil.

Myrtle - Myrtus Communis
Myrtle is a little known skin healer who is a blessing for anyone with open pores. It cleanses and refines the skin, making it smoother and far more toned.

Other uses:
Coughs and colds.

Neroli - Citrus Auriantum
The beautiful orange blossom, which has been made into so many wedding bouquets, makes beautiful skin care. It is suited to more mature skins. It refines the skin, but also gives

it a more plump and youthful appearance, alleviating the look of fine lines.

Other uses:
Clinical trials show that when blended with ylang ylang, marjoram, and lavender, neroli reduces blood pressure. It is also an amazing oil for switching off anxiety. It is not a cheap oil, due to the short blooming season when blossoms are available to extract the oil. You can consider supplementing with bitter orange and petitgrain oils, which are taken from the same tree.

Oakmoss Resin - Evernia Prunastri
Mainly used in perfumery, Oakmoss rids the body of heavy metals and petrochemicals. For this reason, it is used in anything which cleanses on a very deep level. It is now regulated in perfumery as it has been found to lead to skin sensitivity. Use in no more than 1% concentration.

Patchouli - Pogostemon Cablin
This is a confusing oil. It comes from the mint family but smells like a wood from the dampest and most exotic forest. I love it. If you imagine rose as a skin food, patchouli is chocolate mousse. Rich, opulent, luxurious patchouli is a lusty treat for the skin. It pours goodness into your complexion.

I find it useful to use patchouli after sun exposure, because although it doesn't smell like mint, it has that cooling breeze that the mint family has on the heat of sunburn.

Other uses
Aphrodisiac in that languid, "actually I am too blissed out and relaxed to care what you do, take me any way you want" kind of way. If you want more passion, head for Jasmine. It is antibiotic and also tonic to the reproductive system so is indicated for Pelvic Inflammatory Disease. It is excellent for digestive complaints, in particular where there may be

bacteria involved. Patchouli is also sometimes used for treating snake bites.

Palma Rosa - Cymbopogon Martini

Palma rosa smells like rose and is often used to adulterate the more expensive oils. It is different but has equally useful benefits. In skin care, it is hydrating, and also aids skin cell regeneration.

Other uses:
It is antibacterial and also will lower temperatures.

Petitgrain- Citrus Auriantum

Petitgrain is also taken from the bitter orange tree but, rather than coming from the blossoms like Neroli, it is extracted by distilling the leaves, twigs, and bark of the tree. It has a deliciously fresh fragrance which is invigorating and reviving.

Other uses:
Most of the uses of Petitgrain are emotional. It soothes the stresses and strains, alleviates anxiety, and sharpens the mind for clearer focus.

Rose - Rosa Damascena

The fairest of the flowers makes the most effective skin food of any plant in the world. In effect, rose oil emulates oestrogen, so not only does it make our skin look and feel better, but it is also an all-round gynaecological tonic.

Other uses: Emotionally, I recommend rose if someone is struggling to come to terms with grief.

Sandalwood – Santalbum Alba

In some ways, sandalwood works in a very similar way to jasmine and patchouli, in that it soothes hot dry skins, and it is also aphrodisiac. However, sandalwood should never be star of the show. It is a blending oil, a moderator, one that turns a good blend into a really great one.

In Ayurvedic medicine it is used as an anti-inflammatory oil, and many other traditions use it for meditation and prayer.

It is a catalyst for cell regeneration, so if there is scarring, or if the skin has been exfoliated, then Sandalwood will improve it.

Other uses:
Haemorrhoids, insomnia, diarrhoea and bronchitis.

Spikenard
This is an extremely ancient oil which is referred to many times in the bible as "Nard." It is a blue oil and has the same azulene component as Chamomile matricaria. It is liquid anaesthetic, is cooling and soothing, and the go-to oil if you need to put someone to sleep – as in "knock them out!" Spikenard is very powerful!

Tea Tree - Maleleuca Alternifolia
Again, a very popular oil, for its antibiotic abilities. Use it to kill any underlying infections from acne. Zap a spot dead in minutes. It does make a good *ingredient* in a toner, but in its own right, it is too drying. Use just a drop and make Melissa or bergamot the main oil to cleanse and close the pores.

Other uses: Bugs and bad things! Whether it is to treat a bite, or help a stomach bug, think tea tree. If it needs cleaning or killing, this is your oil. It doesn't matter which body system it is for, digestive, urinary, skin, this is your best biological cleaner.

Violet Leaf - Viola Odorata
This is a very exclusive oil. It costs a lot, but you need only use the tiniest amount. It is so gentle and calming. It

anaesthetises sensitive skins and reduces their tendencies to flare up and break out.

Other uses
Because it is so soothing and so gentle, I use this liquid anaesthetic to lull restless babies to sleep. It is an expectorant as well, so it will move the catarrh of hacking coughs. It is one of the most highly prized oils in perfumery, thanks to the love of Napoleon's wife Josephine.

Ylang Ylang - Canaga Odorata
The sweet almost cloying scent of the lily from Madagascar is mainly used for balancing. In skin care, it's used for balancing combinations in the skin, and bringing dryness and sebum production to a normal level. It is incredibly relaxing and will reduce the blood pressure when used over time.

This is also an aphrodisiac oil. Imagine the way a cat curves around your legs, seducing you and bending you to her will. This is exactly the feeling of ylang ylang.

Other uses: Any condition where a set of hormones may not be firing on all cylinders or are spilling over with too much enthusiasm. So, irregular periods, impotence, migraine headaches, ovulation difficulties are all indicated. If you suspect a hormone imbalance, this is your greatest ally.

To paraphrase the Gerard Kenny in his 1978 hit…
Ylang Ylang… so good they named it twice.

Safety Warnings
Essential oils are very potent medicines, and for the purposes of this book I would like to discourage any pregnant women from trying essential oil blends. Motherhood is always going to be more important than the state of your skin. Perhaps consider using the fresh ingredients and omitting the oils.

Epilepsy

Some plants have chemical constituents which are neurotoxic, this makes them dangerous not only to sufferers of epilepsy but also some types of schizophrenia too.

Plants to avoid are: Rosemary, fennel, sage, eucalyptus, hyssop, camphor, and spike lavender (Lavendula latifolia)

Bases and Carriers

To my mind, this is where skin care goes from interesting and quite pleasant to a veritable romp in the most well-decked playroom you ever saw. When you start to understand carriers, you can change the feel of your skin. Experimenting with carrier oils in the same way as you would with essential oils, you can discover some really wonderful creations.

So what is a carrier?

In effect, it is anything into which you dilute essential oils. It can be as basic as the water in your bath or some vegetable oil to create a massage oil. In beauty though, some of your best carriers will be creams and lotions which you have adulterated and improved with your newly gained knowledge.

For clarity, carrier has two slightly differing but distinct meanings here.

We have *carrier oils* which are far more diluted oils which carry the healing effects of a plant. We also have the need to use *a carrier for* the oils, as in something which will dilute them enough to be on the skin. Of course, a carrier oil makes a wonderful carrier, but it is not the only thing you can use. Bath oils, body lotions, and even talcs can all be deemed to be carriers.

Cocoa Butter
The seeds from inside the cocoa bean are dried on banana leaves and then crushed. The butter which seeps out is rich and creamy and wonderful for really deep penetrating healing. Stretch marks, for instance, or really dry feet.

Shea
The secret of the butter nut tree had been lost for thousands of years but was rediscovered about 200 years ago by

European botanists. Despite many attempts to cultivate this fabulous tree in Europe and the Americas, it remains loyal to the ground where it grows naturally, Africa, and in particular, Ghana.

The nuts grow to about the size of a plum and are crushed by hand, then heated and ground to a paste. Water is then added, and the mixture is boiled. The resulting product is what we know as raw shea.

Carrier Oils
The first place I would recommend anyone to go is your own kitchen cupboard, then progress onto the supermarket shelf, and finally onto specialist suppliers.

The oil you use will affect not just the properties and effects of your product, but also its texture too. Get used to feeling cooking oils on the ends your fingertips, and you will notice that oils like olive oil are thick and rich, but sunflower and peanut are far lighter.

Warning - Nut allergy sufferers: most carrier oils are taken from nuts or kernels of fruit. Stay away from oils such as walnut, hazelnut and peanut obviously, but also apricot or peach kernel oils.

Some great carrier oils for beauty treatments include:

Jasmine – This is a bright vibrant yellow and is delicious for feeding the skin. It is well-used in Ayurveda. It is lovely for hot, dry skins and also for helping to reduce scarring. Look in Asian supermarkets for the bargains with this one.

Calendula – This is a cheaper alternative to the essential oil. This is a very caring skin healer.

Hazelnut (*Nut) – Oozing with vitamin E, this is THE best exfoliating oil you will find.

70

Camellia –High in oleic acid, a very beneficial fat for the body, Camellia penetrates the skin easily. It makes both hair and skin gleam with health. Camellia is a great friend to more mature skins.

Jojoba – Use jojoba on skin which has become toughened, perhaps through smoking, sun exposure, or simply through age. It is also excellent for cleaning away blackheads.

Rose Hip – A feast for the skin, it also smoothes fine lines.

How to Make Macerations

Many carrier oils are macerations, which are very simple to make yourself. This is a wonderful way to capture the essences of the plants and create your own healing oils. Essential oils such as rose, jasmine, hyacinth, or camellia, which would normally cost the queen's ransom, can be emulated by making your own maceration.

Fill a bottle or jar with the coconut oil. Actually, any oil will do. Fill it full of plant matter, rose petals, delicious herbs, or potent spices. Ensure they are entirely covered with the oil. Leave the mix for a month on the windowsill in the sunshine. The coconut oil draws the essential oils of the plant down, and soon you have a lovely, magical oil for a fraction of the cost. Some of the world's most valuable plants can be used for not much more than a couple of dollars.

Beauty in the Fruit Bowl

Some of these found their way into The Healer's recipes, others did not. I am a big fan of the fruit bowl for beauty. I'm an even bigger fan of the supermarket clearance section. I buy every rancid-looking raspberry and sour strawberry. Store them in the freezer until you are ready for a facial. They are oozing with the most amount of goodness they will ever have when nearing the rot stage, so don't miss out. Look down the list to see which ones to hunt out for your own face care needs.

Apple
Packed full of antioxidants, apples are nourishing, hydrating, and refreshing. They ooze vitamin C, and so are great for encouraging new cell growth and feeding the emerging cells beneath the surface.

Banana
Rich in anti-aging vitamins, bananas are soothing and smoothing to the skin. There is something very "9½ Weeks" about their texture too. Perhaps this something only the woman of a certain age would get! Naughty, but very, very nice.

Blueberries
You know what? I'm a bit bored by blueberries! However, with all their super-food qualities, they are not going to disappear anytime soon.

Here's the list:
1. They alleviate acne;
2. Smooth the skin;
3. Balance sebum production;
4. Increase circulation to broken capillaries and spider veins.

"I found my thrill, on blueberry hill...." Sing it, Fats!

Dragon fruit

In the heat of the summer sun, the skin takes a bashing. Dragon fruit is a great friend. They are made up of around 80% of water, and thus flood the skin with moisture. It is soothing for hot and sore skins, sunburn especially.

It is also very helpful to acne.

Grapefruit

Most of you will know about grapefruit's fat burning and detoxifying qualities. It is, however, also astringent and tightening to the skin. Be aware, though, of using this directly on the skin, because it is so acidic. It is useful to dilute grapefruit with honey.

Lemon

I used to try and bleach my hair with lemons in my youth, but sadly, it never worked. Lemons do have a slightly lightening effect to the skin though, which is useful for treating scarring from acne. Rub discoloured skin on elbows and knees with the inside of a lemon. Lemons are a little harsh, so use the juice carefully if the skin is already tender.

Lychees

Lychees are great cleansers because their astringency helps them to really slice through grease and grime. The skin is also toned and tightened by their juices.

Mango

As part of the aging process, the elasticity reduces in the skin. That is why wrinkles happen. Mango puts the snap back in the elastic, and so really makes the skin far more taut and smooth.

Orange

Oranges are full of collagen and so are wonderful for mature skins. Use them dried to make fabulous scrubs!

Papaya
When you exfoliate the skin and open up fresh skin cells, the skin looks far younger, glowing, and healthy. There is an enzyme in papaya which strips away dead cells and clears away impurities.

Pineapple
This is a really important fruit to fight the onset on aging. It contains alpha-hydroxy acids which tighten wrinkles and help to alleviate warts and moles.

Warning: Do not leave pineapple on the skin longer than five minutes, as the acids contained burn the skin and cause bleeding.

Pears
I love pears! They nourish your skin and balance excess sebum production too. An excellent choice if you have combination skin.

Peach
If you have dry skin, try peaches. In particular, use the juice for a nourishment treatment.

Pomegranate
Pomegranate packs a double punch with their lovely rich and astringent juice, as well as the rough, hard seeds. They strip away old dead skin cells and then invigorate the blood supply beneath.

Raspberry
Whenever I do a natural facial, I start with raspberry. There is something about the way they change the colour of the skin. (They don't stain the skin, it is more to do with how they affect the circulation.) They enrich the colouring to take away the dullness.

Strawberry

Strawberries hydrate the skin with all that beautiful vitamin C. It is like turning the taps on your skin's moisture switch.

Watermelon

Greasy skins love watermelon, as does acne-prone skin. It is very astringent so it slices through the dirt and grease but it also really nourishes too. The advantage of this of course is you are not replacing grease with oil, but rather, high water content.

Vegetables

Carrot
Very detoxifying, it is also extremely useful for treating skin conditions such as eczema, as well as inflamed skin conditions such as rosacea or acne.

Celery
Using grated celery, or celery juice on the skin really cleans and detoxifies it to the deepest level.

Zucchini
This is a very gentle plant which soothes and reduces redness in inflamed skin.

Cucumber
Cucumbers hydrate the skin and reduce inflammation. They are very soothing vegetables. Those old pictures we used to see of the 1950's beauty treatments of cucumbers resting in the eyes were actually bang-on. They reduce puffiness and refresh the eyes.

Others

Almonds
Bursting with vitamin E, almonds grind easily and can also be brought powdered. Whether you choose to use them in their ground food form or their thick and deliciously rich oil form, your skin will love you for it.

Honey
A super boost of vitamin C, honey is one of the most nourishing and cleansing ingredients you can use on your skin.

Clays
As we travel through the ages of these remarkable women, it is easy to forget that they would have all stood on dirt with its very own specific qualities. Different colours of the minerals in the soils would have different properties. Even still, we have no more than a cursory knowledge of what these clays can do. I'm just going offer up a couple for you to experiment with. Partly this is because they are so very beneficial, but mainly because I love how gloriously messy they are. They also give me a feeling of quiet contentment to know I am not the only person who *cannot get her bath clean*! You have been warned! Wash the bath immediately, girls, or forever hear the moans and groans of your partner.

Clays are incredibly detoxifying as well as cleansing. They also nourish the skin.

Green Clay
Green Clay is the best choice to make a detoxification wrap if you want to lose an inch or so. It is deliciously cleansing and will purge any toxicity out of the body. Use about an ounce (25g) of clay to 1 tsp of carrier oils with essential oil added. Leave a clay wrap on for 20-30 minutes.

Red Clay or Rhassoul

Red Clay is mined in Morocco and is fabulous for tightening and toning the skin. Use in the same way as is directed for Green Clay.

Clay is just about the messiest and the funniest afternoon you will ever enjoy. After much experimentation (because I keep going back for more), I have found that the best approach is to lay a couple of trash bags in the bath and lie on them. The plastic catches the residue and you can just throw them away rather than (ahem) blocking the drain... again.

Precious metals

Throughout history, women have used precious metals to adorn themselves. A symbol that enhances them aesthetically, metals also declare their status to the world. The most affluent, the most important, the most unobtainable... and of course what do we all want? What we can't have. So gold and silver in particular say, "Come and get me, you know you want to, but I'm sure gonna play hard to get."

I don't use metals very much for healing really, but they do, never the less, have healing abilities. Some of you may know people who have gold injections for auto immune problems like rheumatoid arthritis, for instance. Some people have tendencies to develop sores or sties on their eyes. If you are among them, try rubbing your wedding ring on them. The gold treats them every bit as well as the Golden Eye ointment some doctors may prescribe.

Later in the book, I use edible gold leaf in a recipe. I'll leave you to discover which one. These extremely thin sheets of metals are available on Amazon and many kitchen and bakery outlets. They are wonderful for cake decorating, or something a little saucier too.

Gold

It brings wealth and abundance. It instils vitality and helps balance the mind. It helps a person realise their potential. Gold also helps learning.

It has a great affinity with learning disorders and conditions which are "just a little odd." Autism, Asperger's Syndrome, dyspraxia, coordination difficulties, dyslexia, all find an understanding hand from gold for guidance. Rub it on sties in the eye for very quick healing. Arthritis, pneumonia, Tuberculosis, blood and vascular disorders as well as heart problems are aligned with gold. Wearing a gold bracelet or amulet can help to balance these conditions in quite remarkable ways.

Silver

This is very much associated with both mental healing and eloquence. You know the saying "silver-tongued devil"?

It helps stammers and speech impediments. Silver is a very good metal for self-discovery. It helps you to look inside yourself to see who you really are. It is also helpful for people who are suffering from vitamin A or E deficiencies. In this case, silver is aligned to the throat (and communication) so consider wearing a necklace to enjoy these qualities

It also enhances the vibration of the stones it works with.

Copper

This is a useful metal to work with if someone is down on their luck. It enables more positive flow of energy and luck.

It is associated with sexuality and is good for the circulation and the joints.

Copper balances metabolism. It is an excellent treatment for a person who just can't slow down. It calms the relentlessness, supports the body from fatigue, and alleviates exhaustion. Perfect for the toddler who just... won't... stop!

Copper bangles are very popular, with some beautiful designs are on the market. The only problem is... I've never found a way to stop my arm going green!

Precious stones and crystals

In the last five years or so, there has been a boom in the very exclusive skin care brands of the use of minerals to balance the skin.

Apart from the obvious bindi look, there are three simple ways to work precious stones and crystals.

- Use gems in their powdered form to mix into treatments.
- Make Gem Elixirs.
- Create crystal carriers.

Of course, dancing around in the moonlight clad in nothing but an amethyst has powers of its own too!

Not only do the creams and lotions *sound* opulent from a marketing perspective, but also their healing potential is massive.

In truth, no one knows why crystals heal, but they do. Scientists have never successfully proven their properties any further than to say this. Crystals emit electrical frequency vibrations which can alter their surroundings.

And yet....

Amethyst

This is a stone which is mentally and emotionally balancing. It promotes negotiating skills and good decision making. It helps people to move forward in life.

In skin care

It is an excellent treatment for acne. It is also useful to treat skin which is clearly poor due to stress, especially when relating to difficult work or long hours.

One extra tip for those of you wining and dining clients, it is believed if you drink from an amethyst chalice, you will never get drunk. Can you take your own cups to bars?

If any of you decide to make these for a living, strike me up for a sale!

Diamond

It brings protection, love relationships. Excellent for starting new projects, it purifies, and inspires creativity. Imagination springs to life with diamond. Best of all, diamond clears away mental blockages and helps you like yourself again.

In skin care

From a physical point of view, not much use, but from a psychological view point, diamond is very helpful. How many of us hate what we see in the mirror? Dysmorphia, self-loathing, anorexia, or simply not able to see the good points for the glare of the bad are indicated. Diamond is a more healing, rather than beauty stone, if you understand my difference.

Listen to Marilyn Monroe, she knew the score! Diamonds really *are* a girl's best friend.

Emerald
The ultimate cure for a bad temper! Emerald fosters vitality and brings about balance. It helps to bring about change.

Medicinally, this is a very good stone to help with nutritional balance. The lungs, circulation, and immune system draw energy from this stone.

In skin care

This has many uses. First think about balance in terms of sebum production. Skin too dry or too greasy? Work with emerald to bring about equilibrium.

If the skin has lost lustre because it hasn't been fed well enough through poor diet or dehydration, this is a good choice too.

Simply, though, on the days when you just look just a bit too scary to face the world, emeralds will see you though.

Sapphire
This is the stone for the fulfilment of ambitions, making dreams come true, and smashing your goals right out of the park. However, it is not an aggressive vibration. It is subtle, kind, and very gentle. It raises intuition and heightens wisdom. Funnily enough, these are the very qualities you would associate with Princess Diana, the wearer of one of the most famous sapphires in the world.

It is very good for spiritual connection and helps a person to see the beauty in things. Particularly useful, for example, if you don't like what you see in the mirror. It balances hormones, helps aging (as in helps you to accept, rather than stop it happening) and reduces infection. It is a very astringent stone.

In skin care

Clearly, its astringency makes it a very good stone for cleaning and toning the skin.

However, imagine you were a model or an actress, looking for a skin cream. How would sapphire help? Lots of advancement in their career, but far less treading on people to get there. A different type of beauty, isn't it?

Turquoise

My favourite legend of turquoise comes from the Native American Indians who revere it above any other stone. It is sacred to them and appears prevalently, not only in their jewellery, but throughout their culture.

Turquoise protects, and many of the Native American people wear the stones all of the time for this reason. They believe if a person suffers hardship or pain, then a line or crack appears in the stone. They say "The stone took it."

It is the bringer of good fortune. It gives clarity and vision of ambition.

Medicinally, it stimulates tissue regeneration and calms acid complaints.

In skin care

The tissue regeneration is very useful here. Especially after exfoliation, when you have sloughed off dead skills, it helps the skin to quickly create younger, fresher, and healthier cells to replace them. It is also very useful if there is a problem relating to scarring. Cuts, abrasions, burns, cosmetic surgery healing, and even acne scarring are helped by turquoise.

Ruby

This is a very healthy stone. By that I mean if someone is just not right somehow, this is the stone to work with. It balances. It explodes energy. It helps you to find that missing piece of knowledge to make things work. It is passionate, but in the "let's stay together" kind of way.

There is grittiness to the way it works. It can help a person find the will to live. It makes difficult decisions easier to make, and it helps you to be able to accept change. In fact it makes change easier.

It is "in your head" kind of stuff, perhaps the very dark places you wouldn't want anyone to see. Ruby lightens their dark recesses and shows them some light. A bit like blood-letting, I suppose. I have also found it useful for calming nightmares.

Interestingly, the very large ruby contained in England's Imperial State Crown is called The Black Prince.

As you would expect, medicinally it is focused on the blood. Circulation problems, anaemia, blood loss, blood cleansing, and fever.

In skin care

Ruby treats circulatory problems, rosacea, broken capillaries in the complexion, thread vein, varicose veins, ruddy complexions from high blood pressure.

Lapis Lazuli

Ooo, this is the party stone. It is a "thank goodness, it's Friday, I'm gonna let my hair down" kind of rock. The ultimate feel-better stone. Not only does it boost vitality, but it fosters wisdom and mental endurance. It is ultimately creative expression through your own personality.

In skin care

It is more a medicinal stone than one which would be helpful for beauty, but since no-one looks good with a cold....

Use lapis to boost the immune system, and help the throat, thymus and thyroid. It helps reduce insomnia and reduces dizziness.

Ultimately... relaxation, baby, of the let's kick back and let loose variety.

Rose Quartz
If Rose Quartz had a personality, it would be a poet. It is gently eloquent, a bit dreamy, and filled with imagination. It is a *nice* stone.

It is also a red hot skin healer. *Say hello to my new best friend!*

In skin care

It alleviates wrinkles, it encourages more youthful cell growth, and it is detoxifying and excellent for skin circulation.

Quartz
Quartz improves the quality of life and allows you to feel happier with what you've got. It reenergises you. It helps to balance blood sugar and thus is helpful not only for diabetes, but also for obesity. It helps ear infections and tinnitus. Therapists also use quartz for conditions where there is a general sense of malaise.

In skin care

We're back in front of the mirror again here. The key to being happy is to appreciate the things you have, not yearn for the things you don't, and quartz can help with that.

Pearls

Pearls instil confidence and help the wearer to love themselves so that others can find it easier to love them. They are also a tonic for the nerves and adrenal glands.

How to implement precious stones into your beauty treatments

Powdered Gemstones

When gems are mined, they are nothing more than rough stones. They undergo a great amount of treatment to get them to the condition they are in your ring. Inevitably there is wastage from the cutting and polishing, and gem manufacturers sell both chippings and the fine grindings they have saved.

I suppose in texture, I would describe grindings as a slightly heavier and less silky version of talc. By adding these powders into your treatments, you enjoy all of the benefits you would by finding the right essential oil for example. The base you choose to make will determine how you use the crystals.

A moisturiser, for instance, doesn't work well with gem powder, so you would be better off using gem elixirs or charged carriers.

This is for two reasons:

1. When putting gem powder into a light cream, you will obviously affect the texture of the cream (think lumpy white sauce).

2. Even worse, if you use emerald powder you'll look like you are going to audition for a role in the play ***Wicked!*** The brightly coloured pigments of ground gems stain the cream, a

little like henna will also do. Sapphires would also help you channel an Avatar vibe, and amethyst the beetroot queen!

To make a cream work, you need to use either a very heavy base like Shea or Cocoa Butter, or use a small amount of gem into a much larger volume of carrier oil. Then you can blend the carrier oil into your cream.

Here is an excellent retailer of these powders, but you will easily be able to source your own now you know what you are looking for: http://www.mineralien-egger.com/index.php

Gem Elixirs
This works on the same principle as Bach Flower Remedies, Rescue Remedy does.

By placing a crystal into water, over time the properties and energy transfer to the water.

Fill a jar with water, spring or distilled if you can, but tap water works OK. Place the crystal(s) in it. Put the lid on and pop it into the refrigerator overnight. Next day the elixir is ready use.

In fact these are designed to be drunk, and they just taste like water so that's fine, but they also mix well as part of your beauty creations too. Any part of a recipe asking for water can be improved using gemstones elixirs.

Crystal Carriers
Crystal Carriers are created, and work, in exactly the same way as Elixirs, but using oil rather than water. Using the skills learned earlier, choose the best carrier and then supercharge it using a gem.

Oh, and don't drink this one!

One final note on this just in case it is not obvious. The stones you use need not be 15 carat dazzlers. Usually you can find tumbled stones in esoteric and nature shops. Bizarrely, I have seen them dispensed from those kids' sweetie machines too. There is no added benefit from the fire and brilliance of a cut and polished stone. It is chemical structure that is important. Save your pennies, go bargain basement hunting, and save the rest of your money for shoes!

Part 3 The Recipes:

People, you have worked very hard to get here, and I applaud your efforts!

Just a final note before you dive into stirring and creating, and it is this: Natural Beauty is all about going with the flow. Your own natural flow of energy, but also a big element of "make it up as you go along and see where it takes you." Between this book and Nature's Medicine I have tried to equip you with as much information as I could about how to use different ingredients to achieve the results you want. Swap them, change them. Go with the flow.

Hopefully you've had a bit of a giggle, if you remember some of the Healer's brazen remarks but something more than that... please tell your friends. Yes, about the book, but more importantly about some of the secrets you learned about the plants and gems too.

So, without further ado....let's get creating!

For the Bath

"Remember Who I Am" Bath Oil – Mary Mother of God

This blend is for every woman who felt she had lost herself somewhere in motherhood, (perhaps look under that pile of laundry, or empty out that dishwasher. Is it there?) I have made this bath blend for days of crises of confidence, as a way to get back to yourself again. No need for a carrier, simply add the delegated number of drops of oil to your bath.

1 drop Rosemary
1 drop Frankincense
1 drop Myrrh
3 drops Geranium

For pregnant women and suffers of epilepsy, please review the **Safety Data** *before using this oil.*

Cleopatra's Milk and Rose Petal and Myrrh Bath

Whilst there are still a lot of asses about, they tend not to make much milk. Well, you certainly don't see it at Walmart do you? If you do happen to have a donkey willing to oblige, feel free to elevate this recipe with your precious ingredient. The rest of us will use a powdered milk substitute!

4 oz Powdered Milk
1 oz of rose petal (dried or fresh to preference)
1 drop of myrrh oil
2 drops rose oil
1 drop geranium oil

Mix the essential oils into the rose petal, and stir into the milk powder. Store in a jar till required. It will improve over time. It keeps for up to a month if stored in a cool dark place.

Sprinkle 2 tbsp of the mixture onto the surface of the water, luxuriate….and plot.

The Facial Treatments

Hazelnut and Camellia Exfoliating Facial Massage Oil – Margot Fonteyn

2 fl oz Hazelnut oil
2 fl oz Camellia Oil
1 oz Rose Petals
1 drop Geranium Oil
¼ oz Powdered Amethyst

Blend together and massage across the face, using small circular motions. Use the index and middle fingers in a light touch. Work from between the eyebrows outwards to ears coving the whole of the forehead. Gently massage the cheeks. Take particular attention to the chin and end of the nose.

You will feel the dead skin cells coming away beneath your fingers.

Splash off with cold water, or remove with a toner.

Detoxifying Amber Mask – Lucrezia Borgia
1 Grated Pear
¼ small watermelon
1 banana
2 drops amber essential oil
1 drop Oakmoss essential oil
2 drops cypress essential oil

Mash together and apply to clean skin. Leave on for eight to 10 minutes. Rinse away with warm water or a toner.

Nourishing Acne Mask – Elizabeth 1

2 oz Aloe Vera Gel
1 drop Agarwood
1 drop Sandalwood
1 drop Geranium
1 drop Tea tree
2 drops Jasmine
2 drops Lemon.

Mix together and store in a sterilised bottle. Use morning and night. The agarwood and jasmine are to alleviate scarring. Sandalwood cools, and all the other oils work to reduce any underlying infection.

Jessica Rabbit's Carrot Cleanser
Any bottle of cheap cleanser base (Walmart budget brand
work just fine, though plain Castile Soap is nice too, and you
don't have to worry about nasty ingredients.)

2 drops Carrot
1 drop orange
1 drop cypress
1 drop grapefruit

Use to remove make-up or daily grease and grime. Tissue off
and follow by a toner.

Twiggy's Petitgrain Toner
100mls distilled water
1 tsp witch hazel
1 tsp orange flower water
3 drops of Petitgrain essential oil

Apply to skin between each stage of the facial. This will close the pores and further cleanse the skin. Store in a cool dark place.

A Cooling Face Mask from the Angels
2 fl oz Aloe Vera Gel
3 drops Angelica essential oil
1 drop Cypress essential oil
1 drop Dill essential oil

Smear over a clean, dry face. Leave to absorb for eight to 10 minutes. Tissue off and follow with a toner.

Ava Garner Neroli Nourishing Mask
1 Banana mashed
1 tsp slightly warmed honey
1 tsp powdered almonds
2 drops of Neroli essential oil

Drop the Neroli into the warmed honey, and then add the other ingredients. Check the temperature before smearing over a clean dry face. Leave on for 10 minutes, and then tissue off. Rinse clean with warm water, then close pores with a toner.

Elizabeth Fellow

Emerald and Watermelon Mask for Oily Skins
¼ whole watermelon
1 tsp emerald carrier oil
1 Lavender oil
1 ylang ylang oil

Mash the fruit to a pulp, then add the oils to the blend. Leave on the face for eight to 10 minutes. Rinse off with warm water and follow with a toner.

Dry Skin Rose Moisturiser

4 oz grated beeswax
1 fl oz rosehip carrier oil
1 fl oz distilled water
3 tsp rosewater
3 drops rose oil
1 drop geranium

Melt the beeswax in a bain marie. When it has melted, stir in the carrier oil, water, and rosewater. Lastly add the essential oils. Transfer to sterilized container. Cool with the lid off to prevent mould from forming. Put the lid on once cool. Use morning and evening.

Rose Quartz Tranquility Mask
50 ml Aloe vera gel
5 g Powdered rose quartz
1 drop Camomile Maroc
1 drop Violet
1 drop Palmarosa

Mix together and apply to dry, clean skin. Leave on for eight to 10 minutes. Remove with warm water or a cleanser.

Natural Beauty

Rosewater Toner- Princess Diana
50 ml distilled water
1 tsp witch hazel
50 ml rosewater
3 drops rose essential oil
1 palma rosa essential oil

Mix together and put in a spray bottle. Spritz on skin as needed.

Salome's Neroli Moisturizer for Mature Skins
4 oz grated beeswax
1 fl oz calendula carrier oil
1 fl oz distilled water
2 drops Orange
1 drops Tangerine
1 drops Benzoin

Melt the beeswax in a bain marie. When it has melted, stir in the carrier oils and water. Lastly, add the essential oils. Transfer to sterilized container. Cool with the lid off. This prevents any moulds from forming. Put the lid on once cool

The Body Treatments

Exfoliation Oil
4 fl oz Coconut oil,
1 tsp Salt
1 drop Rose oil
1 drop Geranium oil
1 drop Lemon Oil
2 drops Sandalwood oil

Rub over the body to exfoliate and release nourishing Vitamin E into the skin.

Apple Exfoliator
1 fresh apple grated
1 tbs oatmeal
Small handful of crushed fresh raspberries
1 tsp rosehip oil
2 drops geranium
1 drop frankincense

Mix together the rosehip, geranium, and frankincense. Add the oatmeal until you have a paste, and then add the fresh fruit.

Detox Treatments

Hell-in-A Pair of Skinny Jeans
1 oz Green Clay
1 tsp maceration made with dandelion flowers, leaves, and stalks
2 drops Inula
2 drops Fennel
2 drops Cypress

Mix the essential oils into the carrier, then mix to a sloppy paste. Smear over the wobbliest bits and rest for 20 minutes for the oils to draw the toxins into the lymphatic system. Drink lots of water to help the body flush out. Rinse well with warm water.

Lustrous Bosom Balm
4 fl oz Rosehip oil
2 drops rose oil
2 drops geranium
1 drop Myrrh

Place a warm compress over the breasts to open pores then absorb the oil into the skin. It is nourishing and firming. Used to its best effect with the Apple Exfoliator first.

Skin Nourishment

Nefertiti's Shea Butter with Jasmine, Patchouli and Neroli

Mix together:
4 oz Shea Butter
1 drop Jasmine
1 drop Patchouli
1 drop Neroli

Store in a clean sterilised jar.

This blend is just about the most sumptuous skin food you could imagine, rich, opulent, and extremely gratifying. Use as an all over body cream or a hair conditioning mask. Shampoo out and rinse well.

Foot Care

The Foot Balm of Biblical Proportions
4 oz grated beeswax
1 fl oz rosehip carrier oil
1 fl oz distilled water1 drop spikenard
1 drop Yarrow
1 drop Peppermint
1 drop Lavender
1 drop Camomile
1 drop Sandalwood

Melt the beeswax in a bain marie. When it has melted, stir in the carrier oils and water. Lastly add the essential oils. Transfer to sterilized container. Cool with the lid off. This prevents any moulds from forming. Put the lid on once cool.

Make Up & Fun Stuff

War Paint Impossible to Ignore!
Powdered Lapis Lazuli
1 tsp vodka

Paint onto the eyelids for seduction which cannot be ignored. For eye shadow, paint the vodka over the eyelids and blend over. For eyeliner mix it directly into the alcohol to make a runny paste, and paint on with a very fine brush.

Tip the ends of black mascara with sparkles too for that real flash of blue.

For the full Boudicca look, go really red, wine red, on the lips. Nails should be red, but not glossy.

Marilyn's Powder Blush
Simply dust 25g of powdered pearls onto your body using the very biggest powder brush you can find.

Edible Body Chocolate Flecked with Gold
6 tbsp Raw Cacao Butter
6 tbsp water
6 tbsp butter
6 tbsp powdered sugar
Pinch of sea salt
¼ tsp instant coffee
1 tsp cinnamon
Dash of vanilla extract

Decorate with edible gold leaf.

I'll leave the ideas of what you can do with that to your own imagination.

Conclusion

We live on a planet that provides us with everything we need to be well, bright and beautiful. In some cases though, our intellect simply has not led us to find the plants or minerals which hold our cures.

Even as we speak, scientists are investigating corals from deep on the ocean floor and their effects on pancreatic cancer. Minerals have become the stuff of opulent skin creams and the latest craze. And yet, they were always there. Our knowledge just had to catch up with them.

As our illnesses and social diseases change, so will plants and minerals continue to evolve to counteract their effects.

There is such a feeling of satisfaction, I find, in making my own products at home. I am sure you will be thrilled too, when you discover how adapting recipes for your own skin works so very easily. Please don't take my word for it. Get out there in the garden and find dandelions and roses. Substitute an oil here for a smidgen of crystal there. Make it up, mix it up…have fun!

Beauty, as we have found, comes in all shapes and sizes. Perhaps it's the part of a woman which never quite dies. Most assuredly it is the passion in the things which give her great joy. Whether that's her garden, her children, or making her own pots of cream.

You'll never know if this sparks that glint of magic in your own eye unless you try.

I hope you will take the time to read *Nature's Medicine* too (Although it's not quite as much of a "trip" as this particular volume). The ideas remain the same; one plant, many uses. It's a whole new world out there, and it's yours to explore.

Elizabeth Fellow

Check out these other books by Elizabeth Fellow:

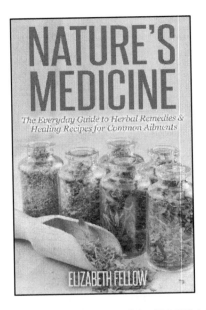

http://www.amazon.com/dp/B00J914MMS

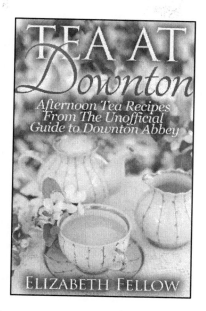

http://www.amazon.com/dp/B00I5ASVX0

Acknowledgments

More than any other book I have written, this book owes thanks to the creators of Wikipedia who helped build the historical references. It took time, but we got there in the end.

Also to:
The Garden of Eden- Jill Bruce
Aromantics – Valerie Ann Worwood